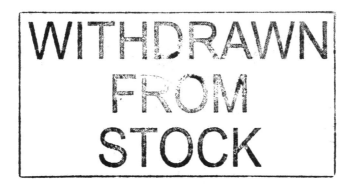

An Introduction to the Physiology of Hearing

Third Edition

The cover images show (background) stereocilia on a hair cell of the chick cochlea (see Fig. 5.6B), and (inserts) upper view of the organ of Corti, a lateral view of the organ of Corti, and bundles of stereocilia on single inner and outer hair cells, all from the guinea pig cochlea (see Fig. 3.4).

AN INTRODUCTION TO THE PHYSIOLOGY OF HEARING

THIRD EDITION

by

JAMES O. PICKLES
School of Biomedical Sciences
University of Queensland

United Kingdom – North America – Japan – India – Malaysia – China

Emerald Group Publishing Limited
Howard House, Wagon Lane, Bingley BD16 1WA, UK

Third edition 2008. Previous editions 1982, 1988

Reprints and permission service
Contact: booksandseries@emeraldinsight.com

British Library Cataloguing in Publication Data
A catalogue record for this book is available from the British Library

ISBN: 978-0-12-088521-3

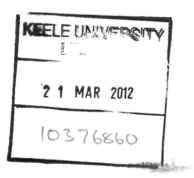

Awarded in recognition of
Emerald's production
department's adherence to
quality systems and processes
when preparing scholarly
journals for print

INVESTOR IN PEOPLE

To Wendy

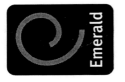

In Fig. 6.21, the two boxes on the left of the figure, labelled CN and LSO, should be clear, and not shaded.

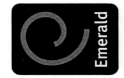

Research you can use

We were disappointed to receive the resignation of the series editors, Kleanthes Grohmann and Pierre Pica, and the advisory board of the North Holland Linguistic Series. We would like to make readers aware that the series volumes "Sounds of Silence" (Hartmann) and "Quantification: A Cross-Linguistic Perspective" (Matthewson) still display the names of the series editors and advisory board, and as their resignation took place before these copies were published this information is inaccurate.

Howard House, Wagon Lane, Bingley BD16 1WA, UK. **T** +44 (0) 1274 777700 **F** +44 (0) 1274 785201 **www.emeraldinsight.com**

Emerald – Electronic Management Research Library Database. Emerald is a trading name of Emerald Group Publishing Limited. Registered in England No. 3080506. VAT No. GB 665 3593 06.

CONTENTS

PREFACE TO THE THIRD EDITION

This book is centred around the way that the auditory system processes acoustic signals. In the twenty years since the last edition, substantial progress has been made in all areas of the subject, and in particular in our understanding of the auditory central nervous system. The chapters dealing with the latter have been expanded; in addition, all parts of the book have been brought thoroughly up to date. Given the rapid expansion in the amount of material available, severe selection has had to be applied, both in the topics presented, and in the references that could be quoted, in order to ensure adequate treatment of the main theme of the book in a reasonable length.

The underlying aim is to show the principles that may apply to the human auditory system. Given that the overriding intention is to show the underlying mechanisms as clearly and precisely as possible, most of the information in the book has necessarily been drawn from experimental animals. For this reason, relatively little attention is given to non-mammals, except where they illustrate principles relevant to mammals and where information can be obtained more clearly and precisely than in mammals. Similarly, mammals with specializations remote from those used by human beings are not included, except where they can be used to illustrate mechanisms more clearly than less specialized mammals. Although substantial advances have been made in the developmental and molecular aspects of the subject, I decided to maintain the focus on the processing of auditory signals, lest the book become too diverse. One small exception has been made in Chapter 10. This chapter deals with sensorineural hearing loss, including current physiological aspects of cochlear pathology, and ways that are being used to reverse the pathology. Here, some molecular and developmental information is introduced.

As with previous editions, the intention is to bring those readers with only a little background in neuroscience to a level where they are able to appreciate current research issues and current research frontiers. The subject is still small enough for this to be possible within a volume of reasonable size; however, the chapters dealing with the central nervous system have, in particular, become significantly more dense than in previous editions. Therefore, it is suggested that non-specialist readers will find the summaries of those chapters particularly useful. It is also suggested that for non-specialist readers, Chapters 5–8 will now function more as a resource for reference than as chapters to be read in their entirety. A reading scheme is provided (p. xxi) to guide readers to the sections of the book most appropriate for their interests.

I am very grateful to many colleagues who have commented on sections, in some cases, substantial sections, of an earlier version of this manuscript. My thanks go to Nigel Cooper, David Corey, Andrew Forge, Peter Gillespie, Wilhelmina Mulders, Dexter Irvine, Matthew Kelley, Jack Kelly, Charles Liberman, Stéphane Maison, Brian Moore, Alfred Nuttall, Yehoash Raphael, Mario Ruggero, Alan Palmer, Edwin Rubel, Jochen Schacht, Trevor Shackleton, Robert Shepherd, Matthew Spitzer, Guillaume Thierry, Eric Young, Jiefa Zheng and Greig de Zubicaray. I am also very grateful to colleagues who have provided original figures, either unpublished figures of original data, new plots of previously published data, or full-resolution versions of previously published figures. My thanks for this go to David Corey, Bertrand Delgutte, Elia Formisano, Anders Fridberger, Rudolf Glueckert, James Hudspeth, Matthew Kelley, Cornelia Kopp-Scheinpflug, Gareth Leng, Christopher Petkov, Cathy Price, Yehoash Raphael, Ian Russell, Donald Swiderski and Eric Young.

I started writing this edition when I was in receipt of a Traveling Scholar Award at the Virgina Merrill Bloedel Hearing Research Center at the University of Washington and I am very grateful to the Board of Trustees of that Foundation for making that visit possible. The major support during the writing of this edition came from the Garnett Passe and Rodney Williams Memorial Foundation, and without their backing it would not have been possible to produce this revision. I give my thanks to the Foundation and their Trustees for the substantial support that they have given me during the writing of this book and for many years previously.

Jim Pickles
Brisbane

From the preface to the first edition

The last 15 years have seen a revolution in auditory physiology, but the new ideas have been slow to gain currency outside specialist circles. Undoubtedly, one of the main reasons for this has been the lack of a general source for non-specialists, and it is hoped that this book will bring current thinking to a much wider audience.

While the book is primarily intended as a student text, it is hoped that it will be equally useful to teachers of auditory physiology. It should be particularly useful to those teaching physiology to medical students. The increasing concern about the extent of hearing loss in the community should increase the attention paid to auditory physiology in the medical curriculum.

The book is written at a level suitable for a degree course on the special senses or as a basis for a range of postgraduate courses. It is organized so as to be accessible to those approaching the subject at a number of levels and with a variety of backgrounds (see 'Reading plan', p. xxi). Only the most elementary knowledge of physiology is assumed, and even such basic concepts as ionic equilibrium potentials are explained where appropriate. The treatment is non-mathematical, and only a few elementary algebraic equations appear.

ABBREVIATIONS

a.c.	alternating coupled
AAF	anterior auditory field (of cortex)
AES	anterior ectosylvian sulcal field (of cortex)
AI	primary auditory area (of cortex)
AII	secondary auditory area (of cortex)
AM	amplitude modulation
AMPA	α-amino-3-hydroxy-5-methylisoxazole-4-propionic acid (receptor type)
AN	auditory nerve
ATP	adenosine tri-phosphate
AVCN	anteroventral cochlear nucleus;
BAPTA	1,2-bis(2-aminophenoxy)ethane-n,n,n′,n′-tetraacetaic acid
BIC	brachium of the inferior colliculus
BMLD	binaural masking level difference
Ca^{2+}	calcium ion
CAP	compound action potentials
CF	characteristic frequency
CM	cochlear microphonic
CN	cochlear nucleus
d	displacement
dB	decibels
d.c.	direct coupled
DCN	dorsal cochlear nucleus
DLPO	dorsolateral periolivary nucleus;
DMPO	dorsomedial periolivary nucleus
DNLL	dorsal nucleus of the lateral lemniscus
DPO	dorsal peri-olivary nucleus;
D-stellate	project *dorsalwards* within the cochlear nucleus
EC	equalisation and cancellation
EE	excited by stimuli in both ears,
EI	excited by contralateral stimuli and inhibited by ipsilateral stimuli
Ep	posterior ectosylvian (gyrus of cortex)
EPTC	electrophysiological "psychophysical tuning curve"
ERB	equivalent rectangular bandwidth

f	frequency
fMRI	functional magnetic resonance imaging
FTC	frequency-threshold curve
G	energy
GABA	γ-amino butyric acid
Hz	hertz
I	insula
I	Intensity
IC	inferior colliculus
ICC	central nucleus of inferior colliculus
ICDC	dorsal cortex of inferior colliculus
ICX	external nucleus of inferior colliculus
IE	excited by ipsilateral stimuli and inhibited by contralateral stimuli
IHC	inner hair cell(s);
I-T	insulo-temporal (area of cortex)
k	Boltzmann's constant
K^+	potassium ion
LD	lateral division of inferior colliculus
LNTB	lateral nucleus of the trapezoid body
LOC	lateral olivocochlear system
LSO	lateral superior olivary nucleus;
LV	pars lateralis of ventral nucleus of medial geniculate body
MGB	medial geniculate body
MNTB	medial nucleus of the trapezoid body
MOC	medial olivocochlear system
MRI	magnetic resonance imaging
MSO	medial superior olivary nucleus
mV	millivolts
N	Newtons
N_1 and N_2	neural potentials
Na^+	sodium ion
nm	nanometres
NMDA	N-methyl-D-aspartate (receptor type)
nompC	no mechanotransducer potentials C
OHC	outer hair cell(s)
OV	pars ovoidea of ventral nucleus of MGB
p	pressure
PAF	posterior auditory field (of cortex)
PET	positron emission tomography
PSTH	post- (or peri-) stimulus time histogram
PTC	psychophysical tuning curve
PVCN	posteroventral cochlear nucleus
Q_{10} or Q_{10} dB	centre frequency divided by the bandwidth at 10 dB above the best threshold
RMS	root of the mean of the squared value,

ROS	reactive oxygen species
s	seconds
S	Siemens: inverse of ohms
S1	fragment of myosin
SC	superior colliculus
SOC	superior olivary complex
SPL	sound pressure level
SPN	superior para-olivary nucleus
T	absolute temperature
T	temporal (area of cortex)
TMA	tetramethylammonium
TriEA	triethylammonium
TRP	transient receptor potential
TRPA1	TRP type A1
TRPN1	TRP type N1
T-stellate	project via trapezoid body
v	velocity
VMPO	ventromedial peri-olivary nucleus
VNLL	ventral nucleus of the lateral lemniscus
VNTB	ventral nucleus of the trapezoid body
z	impedance

Reading plan

Chapter 1, on the physics and analysis of sound, contains elementary information which should be read by everyone. Readers who need only a brief introduction to auditory physiology may then read only Chapter 3 on the cochlea, and summaries of the later chapters. Those whose interests lie in the psychophysical correlates may read Chapters 1–4, and then turn to Chapter 9 (with some specific references back to Chapters 6, 7 and 8). Readers who are interested in audiological and clinical aspects may read Chapters 1–3, part of Chapter 4 (up to and including Section 4.2), and then Chapter 10 (with some specific references back to Chapter 6). Chapter 5, which explores the more specialized aspects of cochlear physiology, is written at a more advanced level than earlier chapters, and if desired may be omitted without affecting the understanding of the other chapters. Chapters 6, 7 and 8 on the brainstem, cortex and centrifugal pathways should appeal primarily to specialist physiology students, although the latter part of Chapter 7 on the cortex (Section 7.2 onwards), some parts of Chapter 8 on centrifugal pathways, and Chapter 9 on psychophysical correlates contain information that should be of interest for cognitive neuroscience.

There is a website where supplementary information is available (see publisher's website).

CHAPTER ONE

THE PHYSICS AND ANALYSIS OF SOUND

Some of the basic concepts of the physics and analysis of sound, which are necessary for understanding the later chapters, are presented here. The relations between the pressure, displacement and velocity of a medium produced by a sound wave are first described, followed by the decibel scale of sound level, and the notion of impedance. Fourier analysis and the idea of linearity are then described.

1.1 THE NATURE OF SOUND

In order to understand the physiology of hearing, a few facts about the physics of sound, and its analysis, are necessary. As an example, Fig. 1.1 shows a tuning fork sending out a sound wave and shows the distribution of the sound wave at one point in time, plotted over space, and at one point in space, plotted over time. The tuning fork sends out a travelling pressure wave, which is accompanied by a wave of displacement of the air molecules making them vibrate around their mean positions. There are two important variables in such a sound wave. One is its frequency, which is the number of waves to pass any one point in a second, measured in cycles per second or hertz (Hz). This has the subjective correlate of pitch, sounds of high frequency having high pitch. The other important attribute of the wave is its amplitude or intensity, which is related to the magnitude of the movements produced. This has the subjective correlate of loudness.

If the sound wave is in a free medium, the pressure and the velocity of the air vary exactly together and are said to be in phase. The displacement, however, lags by a quarter of a cycle. It is important to understand that the pressure variations are around the mean atmospheric pressure. The variations are in fact a very small proportion of the total atmospheric pressure – even a level as high as 140 dB sound pressure level (SPL) (defined on p. 4), as intense as anything likely to be encountered in everyday life, makes the pressure vary by only 0.6%. The displacement is also about the mean position, and the sound wave does not cause a net flow of molecules. The different parameters of the sound wave can easily be related to each other. The peak pressure (p) above atmospheric and the peak velocity of the sinusoid (v) are related by the following equation:

$$p = zv \tag{1}$$

Because the intensity varies with the square of the pressure, the scale in decibels is 10 times the logarithm of the *square* of the pressure ratio, or 20 times the logarithm of the pressure ratio:

$$\text{Number of dB} = 20 \log_{10} (\text{sound pressure/reference pressure})$$

It only now remains to choose a convenient reference pressure. In physiological experiments, the investigator commonly takes any reference found convenient, such as that, for instance, given by the maximum signal in the sound-stimulating system. However, one scale in general use has a reference close to the lowest sound pressure that can be commonly detected by human beings, namely 2×10^{-5} N/m^2 RMS or $20\,\mu$pascals RMS. In air under standard conditions, this corresponds to a power of 10^{-12} Watts/m^2. Intensity levels referred to this are known as dB SPL.

$$\text{Intensity level in dB SPL} = 20 \log_{10} (\text{RMS sound pressure}/2 \times 10^{-5}\text{N/m}^2)$$

We are then left with a scale with generally positive values, in which equal intervals have approximately equal physiological significance in all parts of the scale, and in which we rarely have to consider step sizes less than one unit. While we often have to use only positive values, negative values are perfectly possible. They represent sound pressures less than 2×10^{-5} N/m^2, for which the pressure ratio is less than 1.

1.3 IMPEDANCE

Materials differ in their response to sound; in a tenuous, compressible medium such as air, a certain sound pressure will produce greater velocities of movement than in a dense, incompressible medium such as water. The relation between the sound pressure and the particle velocity is a property of the medium and is given in Eq. (1) by impedance $z = p/v$. For plane waves in an effectively infinite medium, the impedance is a characteristic of the medium alone. It is then called the *specific impedance*. In the SI system, z is measured in (N/m^2)/(m/sec), or N sec/m^3. If z is large, as for a dense, incompressible medium such as water, relatively high pressures are needed to achieve a certain velocity of the molecules. The pressure will be higher than is needed for a medium of low specific impedance, such as air.

The impedance will concern us when we consider the transmission of sounds from the air to the cochlea. Air has a much lower impedance than the cochlear fluids. Let us take, as an example, the transmission of sound from air into a large body of water, such as a lake. The specific impedance of air is about 400 N sec/m^3 and that of water 1.5×10^6 N sec/m^3, which is 3750 times greater. In other words, when a sound wave meets a water surface at normal incidence, the pressure variation in the wave is large enough only to displace the water at the boundary by 1/3750 of the displacement of the air near the boundary. However, continuity requires that the displacements of the molecules immediately on both sides of the boundary must be equal. What happens is that much of the incident sound wave is reflected; the pressure at the boundary stays high, but because the reflected wave is travelling in the opposite direction to the incident wave it produces movement of the molecules in the opposite direction. The movements due to the incident and reflected waves therefore substantially cancel, and the net velocity of the air molecules will be small. This leaves a net ratio of pressure to velocity in the air near the boundary which is the same as that of water.

One result of the impedance jump is that much of the incident power is reflected. Where z_1 and z_2 are the specific impedances of the two media, the proportion of the incident power transmitted is $4z_1z_2/(z_1+z_2)^2$. At the air–water interface this means that only about 0.1% of the incident power is transmitted, corresponding to an attenuation of 30 dB. In a later section we shall see how the middle ear converts a similar attenuation in the ear to the near-perfect transmission estimated as occurring at some frequencies.

While the most dramatic example of an impedance jump is seen with the transmission of sounds from the air to the cochlear fluids, there are in fact changes in impedance at all stages as the sound travels from the air to the cochlea, e.g., in the external ear canal, at the tympanic membrane, and in the middle ear. All these stages have some degree of impedance mismatch with the adjacent stages and are therefore capable of reducing the efficiency of transmission and giving rise to reflections.

Finally, in analysing complex acoustic circuits, it is convenient to use analogies with electrical circuits, for which the analysis is well described. Impedance in an electrical circuit relates the voltage to the rate of movement of charge, and if we are to make an analogy, we need a measure of impedance that relates to the amount of medium moved per second. We can therefore define a different acoustic impedance, known as acoustic ohms, which is the pressure to move a unit *volume* of the medium per second. Acoustic ohms will not be used in this book and, where necessary, values will be converted from the literature, which is done by multiplying the number of acoustic ohms by the cross-sectional area of the structure in question.

1.4 THE ANALYSIS OF SOUND

Figure 1.2A shows a small portion of the pressure waveform of a complex acoustic signal. There is a regularly repeating pattern with two peaks per cycle. The pattern can be approximated by adding together the two sinusoids shown, one at 150 Hz and the other at 300 Hz. The reverse of this process, the analysis of a complex signal into component sinusoids, is known as Fourier analysis and forms one of the conceptual cornerstones of auditory physiology. The result of a Fourier analysis (or transformation) is to produce the *spectrum* of the sound wave (Fig. 1.2C). The spectrum shows here that, in addition to the main components, there are also smaller components, at 1/15th of the amplitude or less, at 450 and 600 Hz. Such a spectrum tells us the amplitude of each frequency component, and so the energy in each frequency region.

Figure 1.4 shows some common Fourier transforms. In the most elementary case, a simple sinusoid that lasts for an infinite time has a Fourier transform represented by a single line, corresponding to the frequency of the sinusoid (Fig. 1.4A). A wave such as a square wave, similarly lasting for an infinite time, has a spectrum consisting of a series of lines (Fig. 1.4B). But physical signals do not of course last for an infinite time, and the result of shortening the duration of the signal is to broaden each spectral line into a band (Fig. 1.4C). The width of each band turns out to be inversely proportional to the duration of the waveform, and the exact

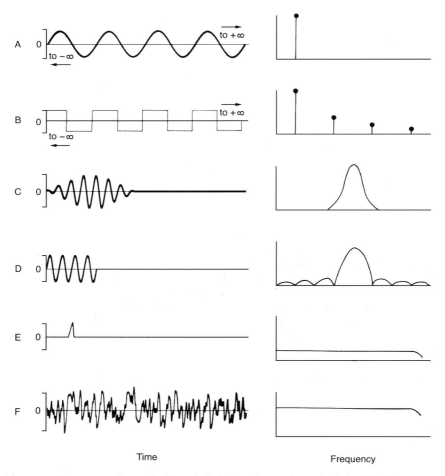

Time   Frequency

Fig. 1.4 Some waveforms (left) and their Fourier analyses (right). (A) Sine wave. (B) Square wave (in these cases the stimuli last for an infinite time and have line spectra, the components of which are harmonically related). (C) Ramped sine wave. (D) Gated sine wave. (E) Click. (F) White noise.

shape of each band is a function of the way the wave is turned on and off. If, for instance, the waveform is turned on and off abruptly, sidelobes appear around each spectral hand (Fig. 1.4D).

In the most extreme case, the wave can be turned on for an infinitesimal time, in which case we have a click. The spread of the spectrum will be in inverse proportion to the duration, and so, in the limit, will be infinite. The spectrum of a click therefore covers all frequencies equally. In practice, a click will of course last for a finite time, and this is associated with an upper frequency limit to the spectrum (Fig. 1.4E). Another quite different signal, namely white noise, also contains all frequencies equally (Fig. 1.4F). Although the spectrum determined over short periods shows considerable random variability, the spectrum determined over a long period is flat. It differs from a click in the relative phases of the frequency components, which for white noise are random.

1.5 LINEARITY

One concept that we shall meet many times is that of a *linear* system. In such a system, if the input is changed by a certain factor k, the output is also changed by the same factor k, but is otherwise unaltered. In addition, linear systems satisfy a second criterion, which is that the output to two or more inputs applied at the same time is the sum of the outputs that would have been obtained if the inputs had both been applied separately.

We can therefore identify a linear system as one in which the amplitude of the output varies in proportion to the amplitude of the input. A linear system also has other properties. For instance, the only Fourier frequency components in the output signal are those contained in the input signal. A linear system never generates new frequency components. Thus it is distinguished from a non-linear system. In a non-linear system, new frequency components are introduced. If a single sinusoid is presented, the new components will be harmonics of the input signal. If two sinusoids are presented, there will, in addition to the harmonics, be intermodulation products produced, i.e., Fourier components whose frequency depends on both of the input frequencies. In the auditory system, we shall be concerned with whether certain of the stages act as linear or non-linear systems. The tests used will be based on the properties described above.

1.6 SUMMARY

1. A sound wave produces compression and rarefaction of the air, the molecules of which vibrate around their mean positions. The extent of the pressure variation has a subjective correlate in loudness. The frequency, or number of waves passing a point in a second, has a subjective correlate in pitch. Frequency is measured in cycles per second, known as hertz (Hz).

2. The particle velocities produced by a pressure variation depend on the impedance of the medium. If the impedance is high, high pressures are needed to produce a certain velocity.

3. When a sound pressure wave meets a boundary between two media of different impedance, some of the sound energy is reflected.

4. Complex sounds can be analysed by Fourier analysis, that is, by splitting the waveforms into component sine waves of different frequencies. The cochlea seems to do this too, to a certain extent.

5. In a linear system, the output to two inputs together is the sum of the outputs that would have been obtained if the two inputs had been presented separately. Moreover, in a linear system, the only Fourier frequency components that are present in the output are those that were present in the input. Neither is true for a non-linear system.

CHAPTER TWO

THE OUTER AND MIDDLE EARS

The outer ear modifies the sound wave in transferring the acoustic vibrations to the eardrum. First, the resonances of the external ear increase the sound pressure at the eardrum, particularly in the range of frequencies (in human beings) of 2–7 kHz. They therefore increase the efficiency of sound absorption at these frequencies. Secondly, the change in pressure depends on the direction of the sound. This is an important cue for sound localization, enabling us to distinguish above from below and in front from behind. The middle ear apparatus then transfers the sound vibrations from the eardrum to the cochlea. It acts as an impedance transformer, coupling sound energy from the low-impedance air to the higher impedance cochlear fluids, substantially reducing the transmission loss that would otherwise be expected. The factors allowing this will be described, and the extent to which the middle ear apparatus acts as an ideal impedance transformer will be discussed. Transmission through the middle ear can be modified by the middle ear muscles; their action, and hypotheses for their possible role in hearing, will be described.

2.1 THE OUTER EAR

The outer ear consists of a partially cartilaginous flange called the pinna, which includes a resonant cavity called the concha, together with the ear canal or the external auditory meatus leading to the eardrum or the tympanic membrane (Fig. 2.1). The effect of the outer ear on the incoming sound has been analysed from two approaches. One is the influence of the resonances of the outer ear on the sound pressure at the tympanic membrane, the other is the extent to which the outer ear provides directionality cues for help in sound localization.

2.1.1 The pressure gain of the outer ear

The external ear collects sound waves over the large area of the pinna and concha and funnels them into the narrower canal of the meatus. Together with the resonances in the external ear, this increases the pressure at the tympanic membrane, which in turn increases the energy transfer to the middle ear (Fig. 2.2A). In human beings, the increase in pressure is a maximum of 15–20 dB in a broad

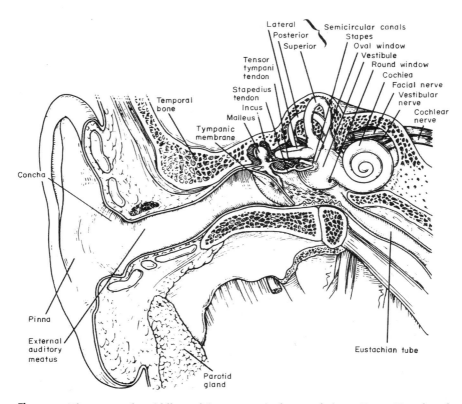

Fig. 2.1 The external, middle and inner ears in human beings. From Kessel and Kardon (1979), Copyright (1979).

peak around 2.5 kHz (Wiener and Ross, 1946). The contributions of the different elements of the external ear can be studied by adding the different components in a model. The results of such an analysis show that the 2.5-kHz peak is provided by a resonance of the combination of the meatus and concha. The 5.5-kHz peak is due to a resonance in the concha alone. Because the external ear forms a complex acoustic cavity, it can be expected that the changes in sound pressure will be highly frequency-dependent. However, it appears that the main resonances have complementary effects on the pressure gain, so that the increase is relatively uniform over the range from 2 to 7 kHz.

Transmission through the external ear is heavily affected by the major resonance of the ear canal and concha, which in human beings is found at 2.5 kHz. This occurs at a frequency when the canal plus concha is a quarter of a wavelength long. This is the dominant resonance of a tube that is open (i.e. low impedance) at one end and closed (i.e. high impedance) at the other, because

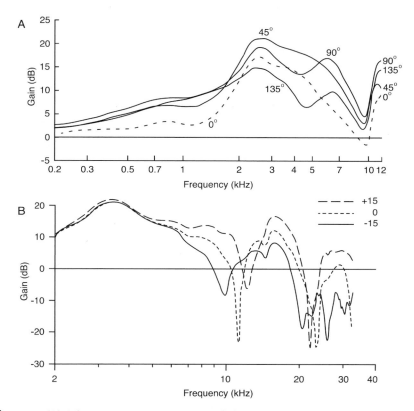

Fig. 2.2 (A) The average pressure gain of the human external ear. The gain in pressure at the eardrum over that in the free field is plotted as a function of frequency, for different orientations of the sound source in the horizontal plane ipsilateral to the ahead. Zero degrees is straight ahead. From Shaw (1974), Fig. 5, with kind permission of Springer Science and Business Media. (B) The change in gain of the outer ear as the elevation of a sound source is altered from −15° to +15° in the cat. Zero degrees is horizontal. The dips around 10 and 20 kHz change in frequency with elevation. Reprinted from Rice *et al.* (1992), Fig. 5A, Copyright (1992), with permission from Elsevier.

then the excursions of the molecules can be high at the open end and low at the closed end. The pressure also varies, being higher at the closed end. Around the resonant frequency, the increase in pressure at the tympanic membrane substantially enhances the efficiency of power transfer to the middle ear, up to nearly 100% in some species. However, the peak efficiency is rather lower in human beings, and in all species the efficiency is much lower at low frequencies (Fig. 2.3; Rosowski, 1991).

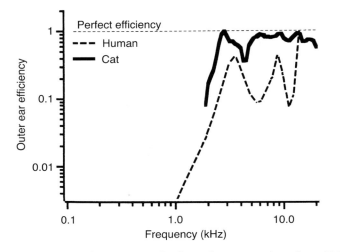

Fig. 2.3 The efficiency of power transfer from the ear canal to the middle ear in two species, according to Rosowski (1991). The efficiency was calculated from the relative impedances of the air in the inner end of the ear canal and of the tympanic membrane with middle and inner ears attached, using the formula: fraction of power transmitted $= 4z_1z_2/(z_1 + z_2)^2$. Reprinted from Rosowski (1991), Fig. 6, Copyright (1991), with permission from American Institute of Physics.

2.1.2 The outer ear as an aid to sound localization

The most important cues for sound localization in human beings are the intensity and timing differences in the sound waves at the two ears. The sound wave from a source on the right will strike the right ear before the left and will be more intense in the right ear. However, this does not account for our ability to distinguish in front from behind, or above from below. The information for such localization comes from the pinna and concha, with the raised ridges of the pinna and concha reflecting sound waves into the ear canal, in a way that depends on the direction and elevation of the sound source.

The human pinna has a raised rim around its rear edge, with the concha giving another rim within that. Waves reflected from the rim and concha will travel further than those entering the meatus directly. If the direct and reflected waves arrive out of phase (i.e. the peak of pressure in one wave arrives at the same time as the trough of pressure in the other wave), there will be partial cancellation or interference, reducing the intensity of the stimulus to the ear. This produces the drop in gain seen around 10 kHz in Fig. 2.2A. Moreover, because the external ear is smaller below the meatus and larger above, sounds reflected from the lower rims (arriving from sound sources above the horizontal) will tend to arrive at the ear canal with smaller delays than those reflected from the upper rims. Therefore as a sound source is raised in space, the trough in the response (e.g. as shown for the cat around 10 kHz in Fig. 2.2B) will tend to move towards higher frequencies. There are further effects; when a sound is moved behind the ear, waves are scattered off the edge of the pinna, interfering with the direct wave and reducing the response in the 3–6 kHz region (Shaw, 1974). It is in this region that there are the greatest intensity changes as a sound source is moved in the horizontal plane (see Fig. 2.2A). Because of the complex shape of the pinna, multiple reflections contribute to the final colouration of the sound, with the colouration being affected by both the azimuth (direction in the horizontal plane) and the elevation of the source (Rice et al., 1992; Pralong and Carlile, 1994).

When the wavelength is short compared with the dimensions of the pinna, the pinna can show a high degree of directional selectivity in the reception of sound. We expect the pinna to be useful in this way only in the high kilohertz range of frequencies. In the cat, the pinna can produce a gain of up to 21 dB in sound pressure at high frequencies, for sound sources directly in line with the axis of the pinna (Musicant et al., 1990). In human beings, there is a broad directional selectivity of the pinna at high frequencies. Above 6 kHz, areas of maximum sensitivity have been measured with a gain of 10–15 dB above the straight-ahead positions, in a frequency-dependent way and over a broad angle some 70° wide (Middlebrooks et al., 1989).

The external ear therefore produces a directionally varying spectral modulation of the incoming sound. In using such a coloration to make directional judgements, we are obviously required to make subtle judgements about the modulation of the spectra of perhaps unknown sound sources (see Middlebrooks and Green, 1991; Moore, 2002, for reviews).

2.2 THE MIDDLE EAR

2.2.1 Introduction

The middle ear couples sound energy from the external auditory meatus to the cochlea, and by its transformer action helps to match the impedance of the auditory meatus to the much higher impedance of the cochlear fluids. In the absence of a transformer mechanism, much of the sound would be reflected. The sound is transmitted from the tympanic membrane to the cochlea by three small bones, known as the ossicles. They are called the malleus, the incus and the stapes (Figs 2.1 and 2.4). The first two bones are joined comparatively rigidly so that when the tip of the malleus is pushed by the tympanic membrane, the bones rotate together and transfer the force to the stapes. The stapes is attached to a flexible window in the wall of the cochlea, known as the oval window (see Fig. 2.4).

A second function of the ossicles is to apply force to one window only of the cochlea. If the ossicles were missing, and the pressure of the incoming sound wave was applied equally to both windows, there would be a reduced flow of cochlear fluids. Nevertheless, in many species the other window of the cochlea, the round window, is shielded from the incoming sound wave by a bony ridge. In these cases, if the ossicles are missing, the sound pressure is still primarily applied to one

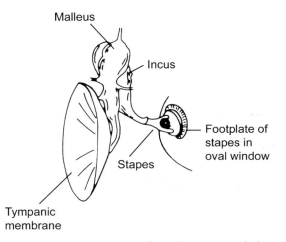

Fig. 2.4 The three ossicles, called the malleus, the incus and the stapes, transmit the sound vibrations from the tympanic membrane (eardrum) to the oval window of the cochlea.

window of the cochlea, and some hearing, although without the benefit of the impedance matching, is still possible.

2.2.2 The middle ear as an impedance transformer

2.2.2.1 The nature of the problem

The middle ear transfers the incoming vibration from the comparatively large, low-impedance tympanic membrane to the much smaller, higher-impedance oval window. As was explained in Chapter 1 (p. 4), when a sound wave meets a higher-impedance medium, normally much of the sound energy is reflected. The middle ear apparatus, by acting as an acoustic impedance transformer, reduces this attenuation substantially.

Following the tentative suggestion made by Wever and Lawrence (1954), many authors have said that the cochlear fluids would have an impedance approximately equal to that of sea water, namely $1.5 \times 10^6 \, \text{N sec/m}^3$, and this led to the calculation, detailed above (p. 5), that if the sound met the oval window directly, only 0.1% of the incident energy would be transmitted. As pointed out by others, and indeed by Wever and Lawrence themselves, while the numerical result may be approximately correct, the physical reasoning behind it is not. Specific impedances are defined for progressive acoustic waves in an effectively infinite medium. In the range of audible frequencies, the cochlea is far smaller than a wavelength of sound in water, and so cannot develop such waves. The actual cochlear impedance is determined entirely by the fact that cochlear fluid flows from one flexible window, the oval window, to another, the round window, with the value of the impedance depending on the way the fluids flow, and on their interaction with the distensible cochlear membranes. The input impedance of the cochlea has been determined either theoretically (e.g. Zwislocki, 1965; Puria and Allen, 1991) or experimentally (e.g. Lynch *et al.*, 1982 in cats; Aibara *et al.*, 2001 in human beings). The measurements of Aibara *et al.* (2001) in human temporal bones suggest a cochlear impedance of about $5.8 \times 10^4 \, \text{N sec/m}^3$ at 1 kHz,[1] much lower than that expected from Wever and Lawrence's approximation.

2.2.2.2 The mechanism of the impedance transformer

In matching the impedance of the tympanic membrane to the much higher impedance of the cochlea, the middle ear uses two principles.

1. The area of the tympanic membrane is larger than that of the stapes footplate in the cochlea. The forces collected over the tympanic membrane are therefore concentrated on a smaller area, so increasing the pressure at the oval window. The pressure is increased by the ratio of the two areas (Fig. 2.5A). This is the most important factor in achieving the impedance transformation.
2. The second principle is the lever action of the middle ear bones. The arm of the incus is shorter than that of the malleus, and this produces a lever action that increases the force and decreases the velocity at the stapes (Fig. 2.5B). This is a comparatively small factor in the impedance match.

2.2.2.3 Calculation of the transformer ratio

It might be thought that determining the transformer ratio would be a matter of comparatively simple anatomy and would have been settled in an uncontroversial

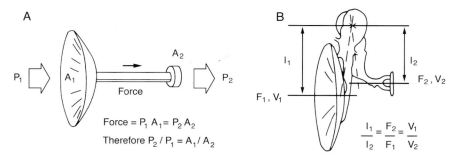

Fig. 2.5 The two mechanisms of the middle ear acoustic impedance transformer. (A) The main factor is the ratio of the areas of the tympanic membrane and the oval window. The middle ear bones are here represented by a piston. (B) The lever action increases the force and decreases the velocity. *A*, area; *F*, force; *L*, length; *P*, pressure; *V*, velocity.

---

[1] This is derived from their measurement of 1.8×10^{10} MKS acoustic ohms, and multiplying by the human stapes footplate area of $3.2 \, \text{mm}^2$ (i.e. $3.2 \times 10^{-6} \, \text{m}^2$) to get a specific impedance.

way a long time ago. This is not so; the actual transformer ratio depends on the exact way the structures vibrate in response to sound. As the movements are microscopic or submicroscopic, and probably depend on the physiological state of the organism, the determination of the transformer ratio is a rather complex measurement. The values that will be used here are those applicable for human beings and are as given by Kringlebotn (1988) and Gyo et al. (1987) (see also Rosowski, 1994).

The most important factor is the ratio of the areas of the tympanic membrane and the oval window. In human beings, the tympanic membrane has an area of $60\,\text{mm}^2$, and the stapes footplate about $3.2\,\text{mm}^2$. The pressure on the stapes footplate is therefore increased by $60/3.2 = 18.75$ times.

The geometrical length of the malleus is about 2.1 times that of the incus (Gyo et al., 1987), and so the lever action multiplies the force 2.1 times. However, the velocity is decreased 2.1 times. The lever action therefore increases the impedance ratio (being the pressure/velocity ratio) $2.1^2 = 4.4$ times.

The final transformer ratio, calculated here as a ratio of specific impedances, can be obtained by multiplying these two factors together. The transformer ratio determined in this way is assessed as $18.75 \times 4.4 = 82.5$.[2]

Does this theoretical transformation ratio give the ideal transformation required to match the cochlea to the air? In order to answer this we need to know the input impedance of the cochlea, a measurement that has been subject to some variability. In human cadavers, Aibara et al. (2001) sealed a tube around the tympanic membrane to apply sound waves to the middle ear and sealed a hydrophone into the scala vestibuli of the cochlea to measure intracochlear pressures. The displacement of the stapes was measured with a laser. The ratio of intracochlear pressure to displacement of the stapes was used to obtain the cochlear input impedance.

Aibara et al. (2001) found the impedance of the cochlea at $1\,\text{kHz}$ to be $5.8 \times 10^4\,\text{N}\,\text{sec}/\text{m}^3$ (expressed as a specific impedance). The impedance transformer of the middle ear will make this appear to be $5.8 \times 10^4/82.5 = 703\,\text{N}\,\text{sec}/\text{m}^3$ at the tympanic membrane. This is rather higher than the specific impedance of air, which is $430\,\text{N}\,\text{sec}/\text{m}^3$. The middle ear transformer ratio is not therefore quite adequate for perfect transmission.

The theoretical value of $703\,\text{N}\,\text{sec}/\text{m}^3$, calculated from the input impedance of the cochlea and the transformer ratio, can be compared to direct measurements of the input impedance of the middle ear as seen at the tympanic membrane. Rabinowitz (1981) sealed a microphone and a small sound source into the human ear canal and measured the sound pressures in the canal resulting from known stimuli. He obtained an impedance for the tympanic membrane of $2500\,\text{N}\,\text{sec}/\text{m}^3$ (recalculated here as a specific impedance) at $1\,\text{kHz}$. This is considerably higher than the theoretical value calculated above. The difference can be accounted for by frictional and other losses in the middle ear.

---

[2] The reader may be puzzled to see very different numbers in the literature. This may be for two reasons. First, the impedances will probably be defined in acoustic ohms (see p. 5). Secondly, the transformer ratio is often quoted as the square root of the impedance ratio in acoustic ohms. Such a ratio is also equal to the pressure transformation ratio. The latter is calculated on p. 21.

Derivations of the middle ear transformer ratio have been a matter of disagreement over the years. For instance, von Békésy (1960) showed that the eardrum in man was hinged on one side, so that it flapped like a door rather than moving in and out like a piston. Obviously, a point near the hinge will contribute less to the total force transmitted than a point near the free edge, and this has led to the use of an 'effective area' for the tympanic membrane that is less than the real area. Similarly, the way the tympanic membrane moves will affect the effective lever ratio of the middle ear bones. In addition, the lever ratio will depend on the actual position of the centre of rotation of the middle ear bones, which can be discovered only experimentally (Gyo et al., 1987).

The transformer ratio was calculated only for human beings and applied in one frequency range, around 1 kHz. It seems that at other frequencies, additional factors affect the movement. For instance, above 2 kHz the motion of the tympanic membrane breaks up into separate zones, and as the frequency is raised further, the effective area of the tympanic membrane becomes progressively reduced, until it becomes equal to the area of the arm of the malleus. This will reduce transmission (Khanna and Tonndorf, 1972; Koike et al., 2002). Gyo et al. (1987) showed that the effective lever ratio of the middle ear bones changes with frequency, becoming largest around 2 kHz, and modelling suggested that this was due to a change in the centre and direction of rotation of the bones at higher frequencies (Koike et al., 2002). Transmission through the middle ear is also affected by factors such as elasticity and friction in the bones and their ligaments, particularly at low frequencies. The inertia of the middle ear bones and their imperfect coupling, in addition to acoustic resonances in the middle ear cavity, will also affect transmission. If we wish to determine the way in which the middle ear affects the transmission of sound over a range of frequencies, it is therefore necessary to measure the transmission experimentally. This can be done by measuring the transfer function, that is, the ratio of the output to the input, as a function of frequency.

2.2.2.4 The transfer function of the middle ear

The middle ear transforms the sound pressure variations of the ear canal into a sound pressure variation in the scala vestibuli of the cochlea. The transfer function can be shown by plotting the ratio of the two pressures at different stimulus frequencies.

Nedzelnitsky (1980) measured the pressure in the cochlear duct of the cat, just behind the oval window, for constant sound pressures at the tympanic membrane. Similar results have since been obtained for the cat by Voss and Shera (2004). Aibara et al. (2001) performed corresponding measurements in human cadaver temporal bones. Figure 2.6A shows the pressure gains for both cats and human beings as a function of frequency. The curves have a band-pass characteristic, greatest transmission being seen around 1 kHz. There, the sound pressures are 24 and 29 dB greater than those at the tympanic membrane in the two species. The responses show irregularities around 4 kHz, but otherwise decline smoothly towards low and high frequencies.

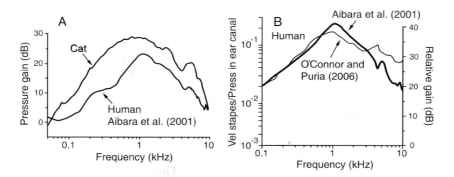

Fig. 2.6 (A) The transfer function of the middle ear. Results from Aibara *et al.* (2001) are shown for the human being and Nedzelnitsky (1980) for the cat. The gain of pressure in the cochlea (the scala vestibuli, basal turn) over that at the tympanic membrane is shown as a function of frequency. Reprinted from Aibara *et al.* (2001), Fig. 8, Copyright (2001), with permission from Elsevier and from Nedzelnitsky (1980), Fig. 7, Copyright (1980), with permission from American Institute of Physics. (B) Transfer function in human beings according to Aibara *et al.* (2001) (data analogous to that shown in A, though plotted using a different measure), and more recent data from O'Connor and Puria (2006), showing much less of a decline in transmission at higher frequencies. In this plot, the transfer function is shown as the ratio (velocity of stapes to pressure in the ear canal). The vertical axis is marked in (mm/sec)/Pa. Data from O'Connor and Puria (2006), Fig. 4A.

More recent measurements in human beings have shown less of a decline in transmission towards high frequencies. While the data of Aibara *et al.* (2001) suggest that the pressure gain at 10 kHz drops 20 dB below that at 1 kHz, further measurements from the same laboratory by O'Connor and Puria (2006) have suggested that the drop is only 10 dB (see Fig. 2.6B). Note that the results in Fig. 2.6B are plotted slightly differently from those in Fig. 2.6A and are shown as a ratio of stapes velocity to pressure in the ear canal. However, this does not affect the general conclusions.

We can attempt to identify some of the factors governing this band-pass characteristic. One factor that attenuates the response at low frequencies is an elastic stiffness. This has been ascribed to an elasticity in the tympanic membrane and the ligaments of the middle ear bones and to a compression and expansion of the air in the middle ear cavity. For instance, as the tympanic membrane moves in and out, air in the middle ear cavity is compressed and expanded, so reducing the movement of the tympanic membrane. The importance of this factor can be shown experimentally, because when the middle ear cavity is vented to the atmosphere, transmission is increased at low frequencies but not at high frequencies (Guinan and Peake, 1967). But why should elastic stiffness be particularly important at low frequencies? This follows simply from the mathematical relation between the pressure of the sound wave and the displacement of the air, and so of the tympanic membrane. Recall from equation 3 (p. 3) that for a constant sound pressure level, the displacement of the air varies inversely with the frequency. At low frequencies, a constant sound pressure will produce a comparatively large displacement of the tympanic membrane and middle ear structures. The forces to overcome an elasticity depend on displacement, and so the forces will increase as the frequency drops. This explains why transmission is reduced at low frequencies.

The drop at high frequencies is affected by many factors, and their relative importance is not known. For instance, Khanna and Tonndorf (1972) and Koike et al. (2002) showed that at high frequencies the vibration pattern of the tympanic membrane broke up into separate zones, reducing the effectiveness of the transmission. We would also expect the mass of the middle ear bones to have a significant effect at high frequencies for the following reason: a constant sound pressure level corresponds to a constant velocity. Therefore, accelerations, and so the forces on the structures involved, increase in proportion to frequency. Further, the ossicular chain begins to flex at high frequencies, also reducing the transmission (Guinan and Peake, 1967).

The position is in addition complicated by acoustic resonances in the middle ear cavity, responsible for the peak and dip in the transfer function near 4 kHz. The middle ear cavities of many small animals are enlarged by a bony bulge, called the bulla, extending below the skull (incidentally, this probably serves to increase the low-frequency response of the middle ear, because it will reduce the low-frequency stiffness of the system). In many animals the bulla is divided into two by a bony wall called the septum. The septum has a small hole, and the two cavities with a small intercommunicating hole form coupled acoustic resonators.

In the mid-frequency range, around 1 kHz, many of the factors affecting transmission at lower and higher frequencies will be small. Møller (1965) showed that in this frequency region it was the input impedance of the cochlea itself that was the main factor governing transmission. He disconnected the cochlea by disarticulating the joint between the incus and the stapes, and showed that the input impedance at the tympanic membrane fell substantially. It is in this frequency region that the theoretical calculation of the transformer ratio, described above, will be most nearly accurate; the transfer here will be least affected by factors other than the input impedance of the cochlea. Therefore, we can see here whether the actual pressure gain observed by Aibara et al. (2001) agrees with the value expected from the transformer ratio, as calculated from the displacements of the middle ear structures. The measurements described above would lead us to expect the area ratio to increase the pressure by 18.75 times, and the lever ratio to increase it by 2.1 times. The product is 39.3 times, or 31.9 dB. This is in the same range as, although rather greater than, the 24 dB increase in pressure observed by Aibara et al. (2001). The disagreement is likely to be a result of transmission losses, in particular due to friction in the middle ear.

Power can be calculated from the relations between pressure, velocity and impedance described on p. 3. Therefore the efficiency of the middle ear, namely the ratio of (power delivered to cochlea)/(power received by tympanic membrane) can be calculated knowing the impedance of the cochlea, the velocity of the movement of the stapes, and the pressures and velocities of the movements of the tympanic membrane. The middle ear efficiencies for cats and human beings

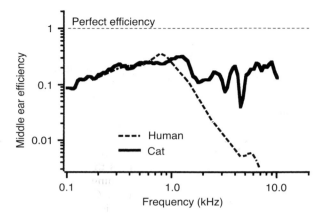

Fig. 2.7 The efficiency of the middle ear, calculated from the ratio of (power delivered to the cochlea)/(power received by the tympanic membrane), in cats and human beings. The data used for this plot are likely to give an underestimate of the efficiency of high-frequency transfer in human beings. Reprinted from Rosowski (1991), Fig. 7, Copyright (1991), with permission from American Institute of Physics.

are shown in Fig. 2.7. The efficiency peaks at around 1 kHz, where the factors described above are likely to be smallest. However, even here, the maximum efficiency is only 35%. The plot in Fig. 2.7 was made using older and probably less reliable data for human beings; the more recent data shown in Fig. 2.6B suggest that transmission in human beings is likely to be more efficient at high frequencies, possibly by about 10 dB. However, even so, the middle ear of cats is much more efficient than that of human beings at high frequencies. Therefore it appears that in the cat, the peripheral auditory system is more closely matched to the input impedance of the cochlea in this frequency range.

Consideration of transmission through the middle ear is not complete without a description of the linearity of the response (see p. 9). Buunen and Vlaming (1981) found that the umbo of the malleus vibrated linearly in proportion to the input sound pressure up to the highest intensities tested (110 dB SPL), to within the error of measurement (5%, or 26 dB below the stimulus level). Guinan and Peake (1967) found that the stapes movement increased in proportion to the input up to 130 dB SPL for stimulus frequencies below 2 kHz, and up to 140–150 dB for frequencies above. This suggests that the movements are linear up to these intensities. It also suggests that there are unlikely to be significant harmonics or intermodulation products at much lower intensities. Guinan and Peake were not able to see any harmonics, although their method only allowed them to detect 10–20% of odd harmonics. In view of these measurements, it is likely that the middle ear is linear with acoustic stimuli in the usual range of physiological and psychophysical measurements. In spite of the linear response to acoustic stimuli, static pressures applied to the ear may be enough to affect transmission, possibly by stiffening the joint between the malleus and the incus, and by stretching the annular ligament that holds the stapes in the oval window.

2.2.3 The middle ear muscles

Transmission through the middle ear can be controlled by means of the middle ear muscles. They are two small striated muscles attached to the ossicles. The tensor tympani is attached to the malleus near the tympanic membrane and is innervated by the trigeminal (fifth) cranial nerve. The other muscle, the stapedius muscle, is attached to the stapes and is innervated by the facial (seventh) cranial nerve.

Contraction of the muscles increases the stiffness of the ossicular chain. As was explained on p. 20, below 1–2 kHz, transmission through the middle ear is stiffness-controlled. The stiffness arises from the elasticity of the tympanic membrane and the ligaments of the ossicles, as well as from the compression and expansion of air in the middle ear cavity. The stiffness reduces the transmission of sounds of low frequency. When it is augmented by a stiffening of the ossicular chain, the low-frequency response is attenuated still further. On the other hand, at high frequencies, above 1–2 kHz, where transmission is not stiffness-controlled, the response is much less affected by the middle ear muscles. Although this seems to be the main mechanism of middle ear muscle action, the real position is more complicated, because there are still some effects in the high-frequency range. In addition, in the cat, the position of the notch in the transfer function around 4 kHz, arising from resonances in the bulla, is changed as well.

Contraction of the middle ear muscles occurs as a reflex in response to loud sound (more than 75 dB above the absolute threshold), and can be elicited by vocalization, tactile stimulation of the head, or by general bodily movement (Carmel and Starr, 1963). In some subjects, the middle ear muscles can be contracted voluntarily without any other discernible movement.

Several functions have been suggested for the middle ear muscles that are as follows:

1. The contraction to loud sound suggests that the reflex might be of use in protecting the inner ear from noise damage. While the reflex is too slow to protect the ear against impulsive noises, if the damaging stimulus is preceded by one that is less intense, but still intense enough to activate the reflex, the reflex is able to give some protection (Counter and Borg, 1993).
2. Middle ear muscles may be able to keep intense low-frequency stimuli near a lower part of the intensity range. Wever and Vernon (1955) showed that the reflex kept the intensity of the input to the cochlea relatively constant when the intensity of the stimulus was varied. This near-perfect automatic gain control functioned for a range of 20 dB above the reflex threshold, and applied only to low-frequency stimuli.
3. The middle ear muscles may also have a beneficial effect on the frequency response of the middle ear. As mentioned above, the transmission characteristic shows a sharp dip near 4 kHz, due to resonances in the bulla. Simmons (1964) showed that the middle ear muscles could shift the frequency of the dip slightly. In cats that were awake and had intact middle ear muscles, the dip was not apparent, suggesting that the continually fluctuating tone in the muscles had averaged it out.
4. At high intensities, low-frequency stimuli can mask higher-frequency stimuli over a wide range of frequencies. Pang and Guinan (1997a), by electrically

activating the stapedius muscle in anaesthetized cats, showed that the stapedius could reduce the masking of a high frequency tone by low-frequency noise band by more than 40 dB. Selective attenuation of low frequencies by the middle ear muscles can therefore be expected to affect the perception of complex stimuli with low-frequency components, such as speech, at high stimulus intensities.

2.3 SUMMARY

1. The outer ear has two roles in transmitting sound to the tympanic membrane or the eardrum. It aids sound localization by altering the spectrum of the sound, in a way that depends on the direction of the source. It also, by resonances, increases the sound pressure at the tympanic membrane.
2. The middle ear apparatus couples sound energy from the tympanic membrane to the oval window of the cochlea. The sound is transmitted by three small bones, the ossicles, called the malleus, the incus and the stapes. The middle ear acts as an acoustic impedance transformer, coupling energy from low-impedance air to the higher-impedance cochlear fluids, thus reducing the reflection of sound energy that would otherwise occur.
3. The middle ear transformer uses two principles. The area of the oval window is smaller than that of the tympanic membrane, increasing the pressure. The lever action of the ossicles increases the force and decreases the velocity.
4. Transmission through the middle ear depends on the frequency of the stimulus. Greatest transmission is produced (in the cat) in the range around 1–2 kHz. Below this frequency, transmission is reduced by the stiffness of the middle ear structures and by compression and expansion of air in the middle ear cavity. Above this frequency, many factors, including the mass of the ossicles and less efficient modes of vibration of the structures, reduce transmission. There are also dips in the response arising from acoustic resonances in the middle ear cavity.
5. Transmission through the middle ear is affected by the middle ear muscles that reduce the transmission of low-frequency sounds. They may serve to protect the ear to some extent from noise damage, reduce the masking effects of low-frequency stimuli on higher-frequency stimuli, act as an automatic gain control for low-frequency stimuli over a narrow range of intensities, and reduce the perturbing effects of middle ear resonances.

2.4 FURTHER READING

The outer and middle ears have been extensively and clearly discussed by Rosowski (1994), who also includes a great deal of comparative information on mammals. Some physiological data on clinical aspects of middle ear physiology are given by Pickles (2007a). Blauert (1997) has an extensive discussion of the sound transformations produced by the outer ear, from a psychophysical perspective.

CHAPTER THREE

THE COCHLEA

The chapter on the cochlea is a key one and forms the foundation for much of the rest of this book. The anatomy of the cochlea will be described first. This is followed by a description of cochlear mechanics, starting with Békésy's pioneering observations, followed by the more recent measurements. A non-mathematical description of some of the theories of cochlear mechanics is given. The electrophysiology of the cochlea will then be discussed, starting with the standing potentials and hair cell transduction, followed by hair cell responses, their relation to grossly recordable potentials, and nerve excitation. Many of the ideas discussed in this chapter, such as the basis for sharp mechanical tuning in the cochlea, are still controversial and will be discussed in more depth in Chapter 5.

3.1 ANATOMY

3.1.1 General anatomy

Figure 2.1 (p. 12) shows the position of the human cochlea in relation to the other structures of the ear. It is embedded deep in the temporal bone. Overall, the cochlea stands about 1 cm wide and 5 mm from base to apex in human beings, and contains a coiled basilar membrane about 35 mm long. Figure 3.1A shows the turns of the cochlea in more detail, and in particular the longitudinal division into three scalae. The scalae spiral together along the length of the cochlea, keeping their corresponding spatial relations throughout the turns. The osseous spiral lamina divides the scala vestibuli from the scala tympani on the side near the modiolus (see Fig. 3.1B). The scala media is separated from the scala vestibuli above by Reissner's membrane, and from the scala tympani below by the basilar membrane. The two outer scalae, the scala vestibuli and the scala tympani, are joined at the apex of the cochlea by an opening known as the helicotrema (see Fig. 3.1A and C). The two outer scalae contain perilymph, a fluid that is similar to extracellular fluid in its ionic composition. The scala media forms an inner compartment, which does not communicate directly with the other two. It contains endolymph, which is similar to intracellular fluid in that it has a high K^+ concentration and a low Na^+ concentration. Endolymph is at a high positive potential (e.g. $+80$ mV), whereas the other scalae are at or near the potential of the surrounding bone.

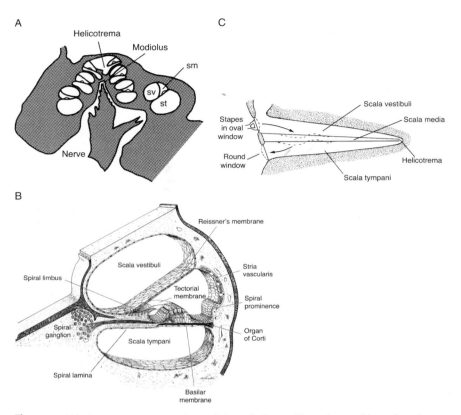

Fig. 3.1 (A) In a transverse section of the whole cochlea, the cochlear duct is cut across several times as it coils round and round. Abbreviations: sv, scala vestibuli; sm, scala media; st, scala tympani. (B) The three scalae and associated structures are shown in a magnified view of a cross section of the cochlear duct. Reproduced from Fawcett (1986), Fig. 35.11, Copyright (1986), with permission from Elsevier. (C) The path of vibrations in the cochlea is shown in a schematic diagram in which the cochlear duct is depicted as unrolled. (D) Cross section of the organ of Corti, as it appears in the basal turn. Deiters' cells send extensions (phalanges) up to the reticular lamina, running in the spaces around the outer hair cells, although they are not shown on this particular cross section. The modiolus is to the left of the figure. From Pickles (2007b). (E) Scanning electron micrograph of a fractured cross section of the human organ of Corti from the mid-turn of the cochlea (the 500 Hz place), oriented as in D. In this specimen, the inner pillar cell (arrowhead) has partly collapsed, and the tectorial membrane has shrunk away from the reticular lamina. There are four rows of outer hair cells (OHC). BM, basilar membrane; CC, Claudius cell; HP, habenula perforata; HS, Hensen's stripe; IHC, inner hair cell; MP, marginal pillars (of tectorial membrane); OP, outer pillar cell; OSL, osseous spiral lamina; TM, tectorial membrane. Reprinted from Glueckert *et al.* (2005), Fig. 1, Copyright (2005), with permission from Elsevier.

D

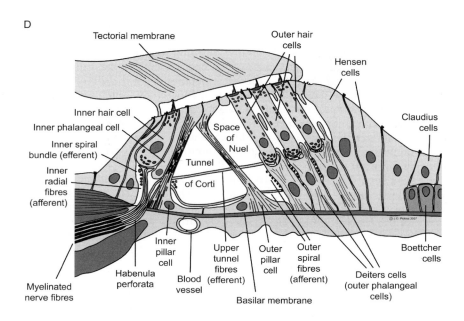

Tectorial membrane

Outer hair cells

Hensen cells

Claudius cells

Inner hair cell

Inner phalangeal cell

Inner spiral bundle (efferent)

Inner radial fibres (afferent)

Space of Nuel

Tunnel of Corti

Myelinated nerve fibres

Habenula perforata

Inner pillar cell

Blood vessel

Upper tunnel fibres (efferent)

Outer pillar cell

Outer spiral fibres (afferent)

Basilar membrane

Deiters cells (outer phalangeal cells)

Boettcher cells

E

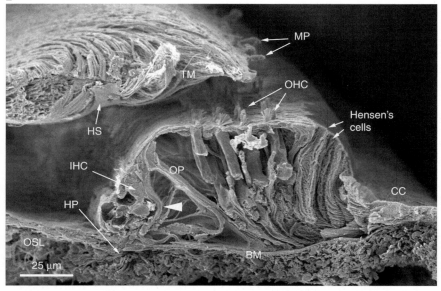

Fig. 3.1 Continued.

The vibrations of the stapes are transmitted to the oval window, a membranous window opening onto the scala vestibuli. The fluid in the cochlea is displaced to a second window, the round window, opening onto the scala tympani. The flow causes a wave-like displacement of the basilar membrane and the structures attached to it (see Fig. 3.1C). It is this that is responsible for the stimulation of the hair cells, and the first stage of the analysis of the incoming sound is performed by the spatial distribution of the resulting displacements.

The basilar membrane undergoes an important gradation in dimensions up the cochlea; although the cochlear duct is broad near the base and narrow towards the apex, the basilar membrane tapers in the opposite direction, the difference being filled by the spiral lamina.

The organ of Corti on the basilar membrane constitutes the auditory transducer and the nerve supply ends here (see Fig. 3.1B, D and E). The nerve supply and the blood vessels of the cochlea enter the organ of Corti by way of the central cavity of the cochlea, the modiolus, the spiral structure of the cochlea imparting a corresponding twist to the nerve and blood vessels during development.

3.1.2 The organ of Corti

The organ of Corti has a highly specialized structure. It contains the hair cells, which are the receptor cells, together with their nerve endings and supporting cells (see Fig. 3.1B and D). The hair cells consist of one row of inner hair cells (IHC) on the modiolar side of the arch of Corti and between three and, towards the apex, five rows of outer hair cells (OHCs). There are about 15 000 hair cells in each ear in human beings (Ulehlova et al., 1987) and 12 500 in cats (Schuknecht, 1960).

The organ of Corti itself sits on the basilar membrane, a fibrous structure dividing the scala media from the scala tympani. Sometimes, though misleadingly, the whole complex is referred to as 'the basilar membrane'. The organ of Corti is given rigidity by an arch of rods or pillar cells along its length, the upper ends of the rods ending in the reticular lamina, which forms the true chemical division between the ions in the fluids of the scala media and those of the scala tympani (see Fig. 3.1D). The arch is surrounded by phalangeal cells, that is, by cells with processes that end in a plate in the reticular lamina. The inner phalangeal cells completely surround the inner hair cells. The outer phalangeal cells, which are also known as Deiters' cells, form cups holding the basal ends of the outer hair cells. The outer phalangeal cells send fine processes, or phalanges, up to the reticular lamina, leaving spaces between the outer hair cells. External to the outer hair cells there is a row of supporting cells known as Hensen's cells, and on the modiolar side of the organ of Corti there is a further row of supporting cells. The distribution of the supporting cells changes in the different turns of the cochlea (Fig. 3.2).

The organ of Corti is covered by a gelatinous and fibrous flap, the tectorial membrane, composed of collagens and molecules unique to the inner ear, known as tectorins (Legan et al., 1997; for review see Goodyear and Richardson, 2002). The tectorial membrane is fixed only on its inner edge, where it is attached to the limbus, although it is joined to the reticular lamina by small processes (trabeculae or marginal pillars). Some investigators believe that the tectorial membrane joins and

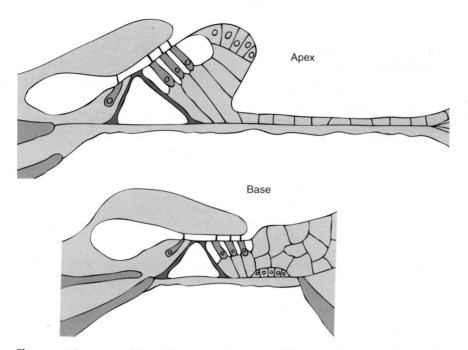

Apex

Base

Fig. 3.2 The organ of Corti shows morphological differences along the length of the cochlea. Moreover, near the apex the basilar membrane is wide and near the base it is narrow. The modiolus is to the left of the figure. From Pickles (2007b).

seals onto the reticular lamina along its outer edge. However, this has been difficult to determine definitively because when the cochlea is preserved for histological examination the tectorial membrane tends to shrink away from the reticular lamina, as in Fig. 3.1E. The longer of the hairs on the outer hair cells are shallowly but firmly embedded in the undersurface of the tectorial membrane. The hairs of the inner hair cells are probably not embedded and fit loosely into a raised groove known as Hensen's stripe on the undersurface of the tectorial membrane.

The tectorial membrane is attached only on one side and is raised above the basilar membrane. Therefore, when the basilar membrane moves up and down, a shear or relative movement will occur between the tectorial membrane and the organ of Corti, with the result that the hairs will be deflected (Fig. 3.3). The arch of the pillar cells (the arch of Corti) would seem well suited to maintaining the rigidity of the organ of Corti during such a movement. Although this appears to be true in outline, more recent measurements have also shown that the organ of Corti may well undergo a complex distortion during each cycle of vibration, as will be discussed in Chapter 5 (Nilsen and Russell, 2000).

Figure 3.4A shows a view of the upper surface of the organ of Corti of a guinea pig once the tectorial membrane has been removed. The hairs or stereocilia

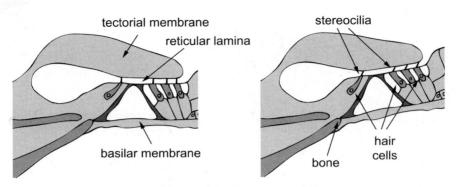

Fig. 3.3 The lever action of the cochlea, showing how the stereocilia on the hair cells are deflected as a result of vertical displacements of the basilar membrane. When the basilar membrane is deflected upwards, the stereocilia are deflected away from the modiolus (the modiolus is to the left of the figure). From Pickles (2007b).

of the hair cells are seen projecting through the reticular lamina, with V-shaped rows on the outer hair cells, and nearly straight rows on the inner hair cells. The geometric patterns on the reticular lamina between the hair cells reveal the pattern of the supporting cells making up the lamina. The pattern is formed by small microvilli, which cover the apical surfaces of the supporting cells, bunching more thickly around their edges. Figure 3.4B shows the relations between the outer hair cells and the Deiters cells, as seen from the outer edge of the organ of Corti once the supporting cells have been removed, and shows the spaces around the bodies of the outer hair cells. On each inner hair cell of the guinea pig the hairs are arranged in three to five closely spaced rows (see Fig. 3.4C), whereas on the outer hair cells there are three closely spaced rows (see Fig. 3.4D). In human beings, there are three to five rows of outer hair cells, and each outer hair cell has three to five rows of stereocilia (Glueckert *et al.*, 2005).

Figure 3.5A shows a schematic cross-section of the apical portion of a hair cell. This is the portion bearing the stereocilia and is the region involved in the initial sensory transduction. The diagram shows the structures common to acousticolateral hair cells, including those of the vestibular system. Three rows of stereocilia are shown in the cross section. The stereocilia themselves are composed of packed actin filaments, which means that stereocilia are more closely related to microvilli, and are also composed of actin filaments, than to true cilia. The actin filaments give the stereocilia considerable stiffness so that they behave as rigid levers in response to mechanical deflection (Flock *et al.*, 1977). The stereocilia are bonded together by sideways-running links so that all the stereocilia in a bundle tend to move together. There are also fine links emerging from the tips of the shorter stereocilia, called tip links, which couple the stimulus-induced movements to the actual mechanotransducer channels in the membrane (Pickles *et al.*, 1984). When the bundle is deflected in the direction of the tallest stereocilia, the tip links are placed under tension, and this pulls open the mechanotransducer channels. In the guinea pig, stereocilia are 2–4 µm long and 300 nm in diameter in the row of

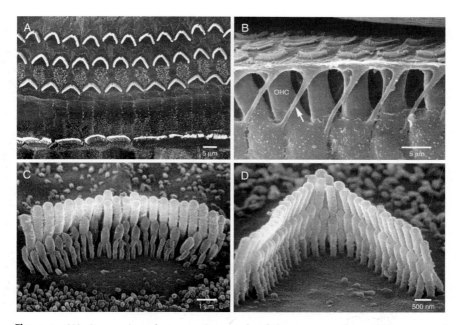

Fig. 3.4 (A) A scanning electron micrograph of the upper surface of the organ of
Corti, when the tectorial membrane has been removed, shows three rows of outer hair
cells (top) and one row of inner hair cells (bottom). Scale bar, 5 μm. (B) The phalanges
of the Deiters' cells (e.g. arrow) run at an angle to the cylindrical bodies of the outer
hair cells (OHC). For this micrograph, the supporting cells on the outer edge of the
organ of Corti were removed, and the organ of Corti was viewed looking in towards
the modiolus (i.e. looking downwards in Fig. 3.4A). Scale bar, 5 μm. (C) On inner
hair cells, the stereocilia form nearly straight rows. Three to five rows of stereocilia are
visible. The stereocilia are viewed from the side nearest to the modiolus (i.e. looking
upwards in Fig. 3.4A). Scale bar, 1 μm. (D) On outer hair cells, the stereocilia form
V- or W-shaped rows. In the guinea pig, there are three rows of stereocilia, evenly
graded in height. The stereocilia are viewed from the side nearest to the modiolus.
Scale bar, 500 nm. Guinea pig.

tallest stereocilia on the hair cell, tapering to some 500 nm long and 100 nm wide
for the shortest stereocilia.

Some of the actin filaments of the stereocilia continue, closely packed, into a
rootlet that anchors the stereocilium into the cuticular plate. The cuticular plate
is also composed of actin filaments, this time forming a dense matrix (Flock *et al.*,
1982). Adjacent to the middle of the row of tallest stereocilia, there is a gap in the
cuticular plate, with a basal body situated in the gap. The basal body is a centriole-
like structure and may be important in development. In vestibular hair cells and
in embryonic cochlear hair cells, but rarely in mature ones, a cilium of different
appearance known as the kinocilium emerges from the basal body. Unlike the
stereocilia, the kinocilium is a true cilium, in that it consists of tubulin-containing

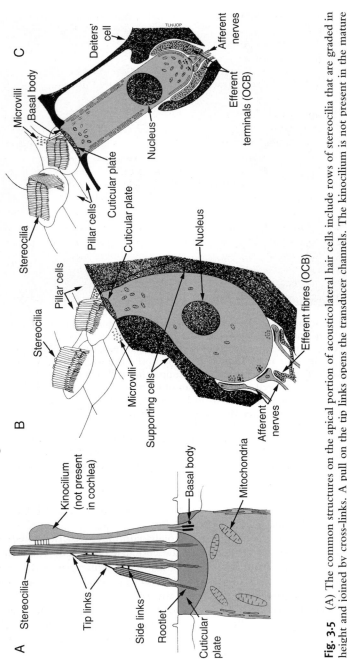
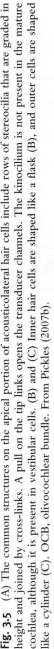

Fig. 3.5 (A) The common structures on the apical portion of acousticolateral hair cells include rows of stereocilia that are graded in height and joined by cross-links. A pull on the tip links opens the transducer channels. The kinocilium is not present in the mature cochlea, although it is present in vestibular cells. (B) and (C) Inner hair cells are shaped like a flask (B), and outer cells are shaped like a cylinder (C). OCB, olivocochlear bundle. From Pickles (2007b).

microtubules, nine pairs of microtubules being arranged in a ring around the outside of the cilium, with one pair in the centre. In the cell body itself we have the usual intracellular organelles and synaptic junctions at the extreme basal end.

An inner hair cell is shown in Fig. 3.5B. Depending on species, it is about $35\,\mu$m in length and about $10\,\mu$m in diameter at the widest point. The shape is commonly likened to that of a flask. The nucleus is central, the mitochondria are scattered, though denser above the nucleus, and the cellular organelles are most prevalent at the apex, near the cuticular plate. The nerve endings are situated near the base of the cell. These terminals are associated with the afferent fibres of the auditory nerve, conveying information from the cochlea to the brainstem. On the presynaptic membrane, the synapse is often marked by small dense synaptic ribbons at right angles to the cell wall, surrounded by synaptic vesicles (Liberman et al., 1990). The synaptic ribbon marshals the vesicles to release neurotransmitter at the hair cell synapse, so that the coordinated release of neurotransmitter from multiple vesicles is able to reliably activate the synapse (Nouvian et al., 2006). The neurotransmitter is most likely glutamate, acting on glutamate AMPA receptors in the afferent auditory nerve fibres (Eybalin, 1993; Ruel et al., 1999).

Outer hair cells are approximately $25\,\mu$m long in the basal turn and $45\,\mu$m long in the apical turn, and 6–$7\,\mu$m in diameter, again depending on species. They have a cylindrical shape. The nucleus is located basally (see Fig. 3.5C). The mitochondria are situated in groups around the lateral wall, at the apex just under the cuticular plate and at the base below the nucleus. The afferent terminals are faced with occasional small synaptic bodies and synaptic vesicles (Saito, 1980; Liberman et al., 1990).

In both types of hair cell, the tallest stereocilia are situated on the side of the hair cell furthest away from the modiolus, and the shortest stereocilia are situated nearest to the modiolus.

3.1.3 The innervation of the organ of Corti

The cochlea is innervated by about 50 000 sensory neurones in cats, and about 30 000 in human beings (Schuknecht, 1960; Harrison and Howe, 1974a). There are also about 1400 'efferent' or centrifugal neurones, by means of which the central nervous system is able to influence the cochlea (counted for the cat; see Warr, 1992).

The afferent fibres, which convey auditory information from the cochlea to the central nervous system, have their cell bodies in the spiral ganglion in the modiolus on the inner wall of the spiral lamina (see Fig. 3.1B). The cells have one process projecting to the hair cells and the other to the cells of the cochlear nucleus in the brainstem. The axons project into the cochlear duct through openings in the bony shelf of the spiral lamina, known as the habenula perforata. About 90–95% (90% in the guinea pig: Brown, 1987; 95% in the cat: Spoendlin, 1972) of the afferent fibres connect directly with the inner hair cells, are thick and myelinated and are called Type I or radial fibres (Fig. 3.6). Each inner hair cell receives 20–30 Type I fibres (Liberman et al., 1990). The remaining 5–10% of fibres are thin and unmyelinated, have monopolar cell bodies, go to the much more numerous outer

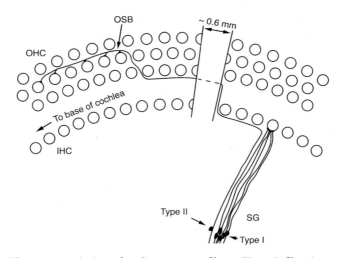

Fig. 3.6 The great majority of auditory nerve fibres (Type I fibres) connect with inner hair cells. A few fibres (Type II) form the outer spiral bundle, and pass to outer hair cells, after running basally for about 0.6 mm. Type I fibres have bipolar cell bodies (i.e. with axon and dendrite contacting the cell body in separate branches), while Type II fibres have monopolar cell bodies (i.e. with axon and dendrite contacting cell body through a single branch). All rows of outer hair cells receive Type II afferents, although only one afferent to one row is shown here. IHC, Inner hair cells; OHC, outer hair cells; SG, spiral ganglion; OSB, outer spiral bundle. From Pickles (2007b).

hair cells, and are called Type II fibres (also called outer spiral fibres). Whereas the axons to the inner hair cells contact the cell directly opposite their habenular opening, those to the outer hair cells take a much more oblique course. They turn basally for five hair cells or so and cross the tunnel of Corti on the basilar membrane, where they are known as basilar or lower tunnel fibres. They then run towards the base of the cochlea for some 0.6 mm, first running along the outer edge of the tunnel of Corti, where they are known as the fibres of the outer spiral bundle or outer spiral fibres. They spiral outwards among the rows of the outer hair cells, synapsing with up to about 50 hair cells, generally all of the same row (Simmons and Liberman, 1988; see Fig. 3.6). However, each outer hair cell also has synapses from several other afferent fibres. The innervation of the two types of hair cell is therefore completely different, the neural connections of inner hair cells showing a great deal of divergence and those of outer hair cells showing both convergence and divergence.

The efferent or centrifugal axons arise in the superior olivary complex of the brainstem and will be discussed in detail later (Chapter 8). The olivocochlear systems have two divisions, known as the medial olivocochlear bundle (MOC) and the lateral olivocochlear bundle (LOC) (see Guinan, 1996, 2006 for reviews). Fibres of the medial olivocochlear bundle arise relatively medially in the brainstem, on the medial surface of the superior olivary complex, and give rise to axons running to the outer hair cells, mainly on the contralateral side (Guinan *et al.*, 1983). Fibres of the lateral olivocochlear system arise more laterally in the superior olivary complex and innervate the region of the inner hair cells, mainly on the ipsilateral side. In the cat, there are about 500 centrifugal fibres to the outer hair cells and about 900 to the region of the inner hair cells (Warr, 1992). The fibres to the region of the inner hair cells do not generally contact the inner hair cells directly, but rather terminate on the dendrites of the afferent fibres under the inner hair cells. The fibres to the outer hair cells cross the tunnel half-way up the tunnel of Corti, where they are known as the upper tunnel fibres, and then ramify outwards among the outer hair cells, showing considerable branching. Near the base of the cochlea, each hair cell receives four to eight efferent terminals and near the apex, rather fewer (Liberman *et al.*, 1990). The efferent terminals are large and vesiculated and tend to surround the base of the cell and its afferent terminals.

The cochlea also receives an adrenergic, sympathetic innervation (Densert and Flock, 1974; Vicente-Torres and Gil-Loyzaga, 2002). Most of the fibres appear to end on blood vessels in the spiral lamina. Others appear to terminate near the afferent nerve fibres as they pass through the habenula perforata. There are also adrenergic receptors in the stria vascularis, on the inner and outer hair cells and on the cell bodies of the cochlear nerve fibres, i.e. the spiral ganglion cells that would be capable of responding to circulating adrenaline (Fauser *et al.*, 2004).

3.2 THE MECHANICS OF THE COCHLEA

3.2.1 The travelling wave

When a sound impinges on the eardrum, the vibrations are transmitted to the oval window by the middle ear bones. The vibrations then cause a movement of the cochlear fluids and the cochlear partitions, displacing the fluid to the round window (see Fig. 3.1C). This initiates a wave of displacement on the basilar membrane, which then travels apically in the cochlea. The wave is a very important stage in the analysis of sound by the auditory system, because the pattern and position of the wave depends on the frequency of the stimulus. For a sine wave of a single frequency, the vibration has a sharp peak which is confined to a narrow region of the basilar membrane. Moreover, the position of the peak depends on the frequency of the stimulus. The mechanical analysis of frequency by the cochlea underlies the frequency selectivity shown by the later stages of the auditory system and the selectivity that can be shown psychophysically. The frequency selectivity depends on the physical mechanics of the basilar membrane and the cochlear fluids, and their interaction with physiological hair cell responses. The most recent results are a development of the approach pioneered by G. von Békésy, and a discussion of his results still provides the best way of introducing the current work.

Békésy in a long series of experiments, described in a collected form by Békésy (1960), examined the movement of the cochlear partition in human and animal cadavers. Temporal bones were rapidly dissected soon after death and were immersed in saline solution. Rubber windows were substituted for the round and oval windows, and a mechanical vibrator was attached to one of them. The cochlear wall was opened under water for observation of the partitions within. By microscopic and stroboscopic observation of silver particles scattered on Reissner's membrane, Békésy was able to plot out the now-classic travelling wave pattern shown in Fig. 3.7. He presumed that this was similar to the movement of the membrane carrying the transducers themselves, namely the basilar membrane. For a stimulus of fixed frequency, the cochlear partition vibrated with a wave that gradually grew in amplitude as it moved up the cochlea from the stapes, reached a maximum, and then rapidly declined. The wave of displacement moved more and more slowly as it passed up the cochlea, so the phase changed with distance at an accelerating rate and the apparent wavelength of the vibration decreased. However, the frequency of vibration at any point was, of course, the same as that of the input.

Békésy's plots were made in two ways. By opening a length of cochlea, it was possible to see the pattern of movement distributed along the membrane, and so plot the waveforms and their envelopes for sounds of different frequencies. The vibration envelopes found by Békésy are shown in Fig. 3.8. They show the important point that as the frequency of the stimulus was increased, the position of the vibration maximum moved towards the base of the cochlea. Thus high-frequency tones produced a vibration pattern peaking at the base of the cochlea. Low-frequency tones, in contrast, produced most vibration in the apex of the cochlea, although, because of the long tail of the vibration envelope, there was some response near the base as well.

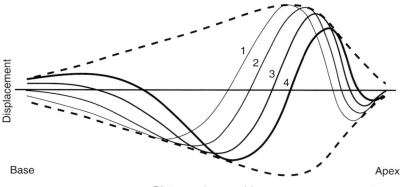

Fig. 3.7 Travelling waves in the cochlea were first shown by Békésy. The full lines show the pattern of the deflection of the cochlear partition at successive instants, as numbered. The waves are contained within an envelope that is static (dotted lines). Stimulus frequency, 200 Hz. Reprinted from Békésy (1953), Fig. 22, Copyright (1953), with permission from American Institute of Physics.

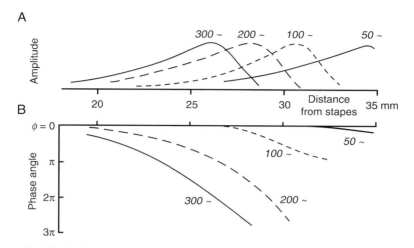

Fig. 3.8 (A) Displacement envelopes on the cochlear partition are shown for tones of different frequencies. (B) The relative phase angle of the displacement. Reprinted from Békésy (1947), Fig. 5, Copyright (1947), with permission from American Institute of Physics.

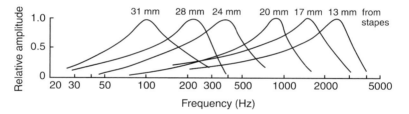

Fig. 3.9 Frequency responses are shown for six different points on the cochlear partition. The amplitude of the travelling wave envelope was measured as the stimulus frequency was varied with constant peak stapes displacements. The position of the point of observation is marked on each curve. Reprinted from Békésy (1949), Fig. 7, Copyright (1949), with permission from American Institute of Physics.

A second way in which Békésy measured the vibration pattern is indicated in Fig. 3.9. He opened the cochlea at certain points and measured the vibration at those points as the frequency was varied. Figure 3.9 shows his results for six points on the membrane, the peak-to-peak stapes displacement being kept constant as he varied the frequency at each point. Note that, as before, it is the most basal point that responds best to the highest frequencies. Note the shallow slope on the low-frequency side and the much steeper slope on the high-frequency side. In going from the space axis of Fig. 3.8 to the frequency axis of Fig. 3.9, the direction of variation of the parameters marked on the curves and the abscissa have to be reversed, although the positions of the steep and shallow slopes are the same.

of this intensity, the cochlea is sharply tuned, because changing the stimulus frequency by only a little produces a large change in the amplitude of vibration. The basilar membrane therefore shows a *band-pass* filter function, with a high degree of frequency selectivity.

At higher intensities of stimulation, the sharp tuning disappears (e.g. at 90 dB SPL). The response now shows only a broad peak. Not only does the pattern spread preferentially in the low-frequency direction, but also the frequency giving the maximum response moves towards lower frequencies. This occurs because as the stimulus intensity is raised, the response grows only slowly in the region of the peak, and faster for lower frequencies of stimulation.

Figure 3.11B shows the same data plotted as tuning curves, or frequency-threshold curves (FTCs). The graph shows the relations between stimulus frequency and stimulus intensity necessary to produce certain criterion, amplitudes or velocities of vibration. The lowest curve, like the lowest curve in Fig. 3.11A, shows that the system is very sensitive at one frequency, 10 kHz, and very sharply tuned. This frequency is known as the *characteristic frequency* (CF) of the place or nerve fibre being measured. The basilar membrane is sensitive because at 10 kHz a response of the lowest criterion amplitude (0.4 nm) is produced by a stimulus intensity of only 13 dB SPL. It is sharply tuned because if the stimulus frequency is moved away from 10 kHz, the stimulus intensity has to be increased markedly to produce the same criterion response. An advantage of presenting the data in this way is that it is possible to compare directly the tuning from different stages of the auditory system. For instance, if we go through a similar procedure and construct a tuning curve for an auditory nerve fibre innervating the same region of the cochlea, using as our criterion a certain number of evoked action potentials per second, we obtain a tuning curve that is similar in general shape to the mechanical ones (thick solid line, Fig. 3.11B). This shows that the tuning of the auditory nerve fibres matches, to a first approximation at least, the tuning of the basilar membrane.

The plots in Fig. 3.10, with distance on the horizontal axis, and those in Fig. 3.11, with frequency on the horizontal axis, are equivalent representations of the same data. They can be calculated from each other as long as we know how the position of the peak of the travelling wave depends on the frequency of the stimulus and how the shape of the travelling wave changes for different frequencies of stimulation. Figure 3.12 shows how the plots are interrelated. It is a useful exercise for the reader to become practiced in understanding the relation between the two representations so that he or she can immediately understand the implications in the spatial domain of data presented in the frequency domain, and vice versa.

3.2.2.4 Non-linearity of the response

Figures 3.10B and 3.11A show that as the stimulus intensity is raised, the amplitude of the response can grow non-linearly, i.e. it can grow less than in proportion to the increase in stimulus intensity. This compressive non-linearity is particularly visible near the peak of the travelling wave (arrow, Fig. 3.10B), or in frequency plots at the characteristic frequency (arrow, Fig. 3.11A).

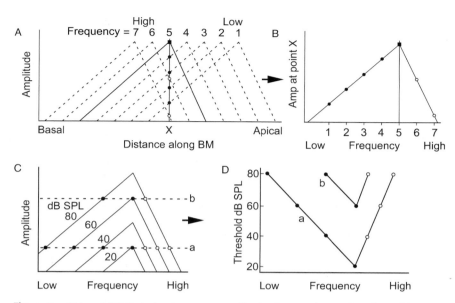

Fig. 3.12 (A) and (B) Relation between amplitude plots made as a function of distance (A) and amplitude plots made as a function of frequency (B). Full and dotted lines in A show responses for different frequencies of stimulation. Frequency 7 is high and frequency 1 is low. The plot in B can be derived from the data in A, by looking at the amplitude of the response at one point (×) on the basilar membrane. Closed circles show data derived from frequencies of stimulation below that giving the maximum response at point × and open circles from frequencies above. It is also possible to construct the plots in A from the plot in B, if the place–frequency map is known, i.e. if the relation between the position of the peak of the travelling wave and the frequency of stimulation is known, and if the change in shape of the travelling wave with change in frequency is known. It is generally a reasonable assumption that for small changes in frequency, the travelling wave maintains the same overall shape as it changes in position. (C and D) Construction of tuning curves from amplitude–frequency plots. (C) Amplitudes of response as a function of frequency, for different intensities of stimulation (dB SPL marked on curves). Tuning curves in D are shown for two amplitude criteria (a and b).

The non-linearity is shown more explicitly in the amplitude plots of Fig. 3.13. In Fig. 3.13A, the amplitude of the basilar membrane vibration is shown for different amplitudes and frequencies of stimulation. At the characteristic frequency, 10 kHz, the response increases approximately linearly with intensity until about 20 dB SPL and then increases with a slope of about 0.3 (on log–log axes). Higher frequencies of stimulation (e.g. 11 kHz) show a similar non-linearity. However, at frequencies well below the characteristic frequency, the non-linearity is reduced or absent. After death (p.m., at 9 kHz) the cochlea becomes much less sensitive and the response becomes linear.

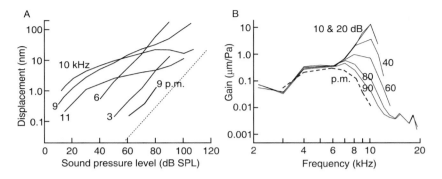

Fig. 3.13 The non-linearity of basilar membrane vibration. (A) Magnitude of basilar membrane vibration is shown as a function of stimulus intensity (horizontal scale) and for different frequencies of stimulation (as marked on curves, in kHz). The heavy dotted line marked p.m. was measured after death (at stimulus frequency 9 kHz). The graph has log–log axes, because the decibel scale uses a logarithmic transformation of stimulus intensity. The fine dotted line has a slope of 1, i.e. as for linear growth. Near and above the characteristic frequency (near and above 10 kHz), and for stimulus intensities above 20–30 dB SPL, the slope of the intensity functions is less than 1, i.e. the responses show a compressive non-linearity. At lower frequencies, the slope is 1 or near 1. After death, the cochlea loses sensitivity and the response becomes linear. Data recalculated from Ruggero *et al.* (1997). (B) The data of Fig. 3.11A, replotted as a gain (i.e. amplitude of displacement divided by stimulus intensity) and shown as a frequency response. The intensity of stimulation (in dB SPL) is marked on the curves. The dotted line marked p.m. was measured after death. Data recalculated from Ruggero *et al.* (1997) and from Recio *et al.* (1998) (post-mortem).

In Fig. 3.13B, the response is plotted as a gain, i.e. as response amplitude divided by stimulus amplitude, as a function of frequency. If the responses were entirely linear, all curves would lie on top of each other. Figure 3.13B shows how the gain of the basilar membrane response is greatest around the characteristic frequency, and at the lowest intensities of stimulation (e.g. 10 and 20 dB SPL). At the highest intensity of stimulation (90 dB SPL), the gain is much lower, and after death the gain is a little lower still (p.m., dotted line). The pattern of vibration is now similar to the insensitive, broadly tuned and substantially low-pass filter response, originally found by Békésy.

This gives a hint as to the mechanism behind sharp tuning and suggests that when the cochlea is in good physiological condition, a sensitive and sharply tuned component of the response is added to an insensitive and broadly tuned component. The sensitive component disappears when the cochlea is in a poor condition.

The most widely accepted hypothesis for the production of the sharply tuned tip in the tuning curve is a rather surprising and revolutionary one. The hypothesis says that the cochlea contains an *active mechanical amplifier*. The amplifier is triggered by the acoustic stimulus and feeds mechanical energy back into the travelling wave, thus increasing the amplitude of the vibration. It also produces the sharply tuned response. The mechanism of this mechanical amplification is still controversial, and some of the thinking behind the hypotheses will be described in Section 3.2.3 when theories of cochlear mechanics are discussed. However, a more detailed consideration of the evidence will be delayed until Chapter 5. Here, we note that the presence of a mechanically active factor in cochlear mechanics could explain the extreme physiological vulnerability of the low-threshold, sharply tuned component of the travelling wave.

The non-linearity also has a very important functional consequence, because it allows the discrimination of auditory stimuli over a very wide (120 dB) range of stimulus intensities.

3.2.2.5 Phase of the response

Because the travelling wave moves from base to apex, its phase increases with distance along the cochlear duct. This was shown by Békésy (see Fig. 3.8B) and has been confirmed by more recent measurements. Figure 3.14A shows the phase

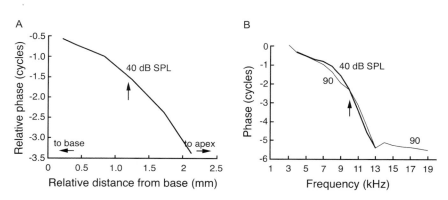

Fig. 3.14 Phase of basilar membrane response (dB SPL marked on curves). Phase lags at the measuring point are plotted downwards. (A) Phase of basilar membrane response to a 10-kHz tone, as a function of relative (not absolute) distance along the basilar membrane, in the chinchilla cochlea. The vertical arrow shows the position of the peak of the travelling wave. The wave shows increasing phase lag as it moves towards the apex of the cochlea. Reprinted from Rhode and Recio (2000), Fig. 5D, Copyright (2000), with permission from American Institute of Physics. (B) Phase of response, at a single point 3.5 mm from the base of the chinchilla cochlea, as a function of frequency of stimulation. The vertical arrow shows the characteristic frequency of the point being measured (10 kHz). Note difference in vertical scale from part A. Measurements were made at two different stimulus intensities (40 and 90 dB SPL). Phase = 0 means that displacement to scala tympani is in phase with low pressure at the eardrum. Reprinted from Ruggero et al. (1997), Fig. 13, Copyright (1997), with permission from American Institute of Physics.

response to a tone of fixed frequency, as a function of distance, and demonstrates a similar increase in phase with distance from the cochlear base. With this technique, the spatial restrictions of the window into the cochlea did not permit the observation of the whole length of the travelling wave and therefore the total phase change accumulated by the travelling wave along its whole length could not be measured. An alternative method is shown in Fig. 3.14B. Here, the observation is made at a single point, and the frequency of stimulation is varied. This sweeps the whole travelling wave across the point of observation, permitting the total phase shift of a wave to be measured.

The phase data show that there are three regions in the travelling wave. The phase curve has a shallow slope towards the left of Fig. 3.14A. This means that here the phase of the wave increases only a little with distance along the duct, which means that the wave travels relatively rapidly over the first part of the cochlear duct. Near the peak of the travelling wave (arrow in Fig. 3.14A), the phase increases more rapidly with distance, meaning that the wave moves more slowly as it travels through this region. We note that at the peak of the travelling wave, the total phase shift is approximately 2–3 cycles (shown in the frequency response, in Fig. 3.14B), though this varies with species, frequency region, and investigator. Well beyond the peak of the travelling wave, when the wave has become very small, the phase response becomes essentially flat (Fig. 3.14B). This means that the whole apical region of the cochlea beyond the region where the travelling wave is developed, known as the 'plateau region', vibrates in phase, though admittedly at a very small amplitude.

3.2.3 Theories of cochlear mechanics

The vibration of the cochlear partition has been investigated theoretically, initially by means of mechanical models, and more recently mathematically, through analytic approaches or with computer models. There seems to be a satisfactory explanation of the broadly tuned wave that is seen in cochleae in poor physiological condition. This will be described first. The basis of the sensitive and sharply tuned component of the wave, seen in cochleae in good physiological condition, is more controversial, and some ideas will be discussed later. The issues discussed here will be dealt with in greater detail in Chapter 5.

3.2.3.1 The broadly tuned component of the travelling wave: passive cochlear mechanics

A consensus seems to be emerging about the physical basis of the broadly tuned component of the travelling wave (see, e.g., de Boer, 1996; Patuzzi, 1996; Robles and Ruggero, 2001). In the most general terms, the wave is analogous to a wave on the surface of water. In such a water wave, once the energy is introduced, it is carried passively along the wave by the inertia of fluid motion in the horizontal direction. Gravity provides the restoring forces in the vertical direction. The passive cochlear wave is similar, except that the restoring forces come from the stiffness of the cochlear partition (i.e. from the stiffness of the basilar membrane and all its associated structures, such as the organ of Corti and the tectorial membrane). The inertial forces include a component from the mass of the cochlear partition, as well as from the mass of the fluid. Theories are expressed in terms of either shallow-water waves (also known as long waves) in which the wavelength is long compared to the depth of the cochlear duct, or deep-water waves (also known as short waves) in which the wavelength is short compared to the depth of the cochlear duct. While the rather simpler long-wave analysis is possible well basal to the peak of the travelling wave, the wavelength becomes short near the peak, and here a short-wave analysis is necessary.

The passive cochlear travelling wave differs from a water surface wave in two respects. Firstly, it always travels from base to apex of the cochlea, whereas a water wave radiates away from the source in all directions. Secondly, the cochlear travelling wave has a particular dependence on the distance of travel along the cochlea, since unlike a water wave it grows in amplitude as it passes down the cochlea, comes to a maximum, and then declines sharply, with the position of the peak depending on the stimulus frequency. The different behaviour in these two respects is a result of the variation in the stiffness of the cochlear partition from base to apex.

It was originally shown by Békésy, and more recently confirmed by Emadi *et al.* (2004), that the cochlear partition is relatively stiff near the base and relatively compliant near the apex. This affects the way that the partition vibrates in response to sound. Near the base, where the stiffness is high, stiffness is the most important factor governing the vibration of the partition. Vibrations here are known as stiffness-limited. Towards the apex, where the stiffness is lower, the masses and inertias of the system instead limit the vibration, and the vibration is known as mass-limited. In response to an applied force, a stiffness-limited system will always start to move before a mass-limited one. This means that when a pressure difference is applied across any small segment of the cochlear partition, the more stiffness-limited part towards the base will move first followed by the more mass-limited part towards the apex. A wave of deflection therefore travels up the cochlea, from base to apex, the direction depending only on the gradation of compliance and not how the pressure difference is introduced.

The relative delay in the movement of the more apical portion induces longitudinal flow of the fluid, and the inertia of this flow carries the energy towards the apex. The travelling wave therefore primarily depends on the interaction between the stiffness of the partition in response to deflection and the inertia of fluid moving along the duct.

Why does the travelling wave grow in amplitude as it passes up the duct, and why is there a peak in the vibration? In order to answer this, we need to know more about how the mechanical properties of the cochlear partition vary along the duct.

Firstly, the partition becomes less stiff towards the apex so that a certain pressure difference across the partition will induce greater amplitudes of movement towards the apex. This is shown in the plot of the admittance of the membrane in Fig. 3.15A, where on the left of the diagram, for the stiffness-limited region

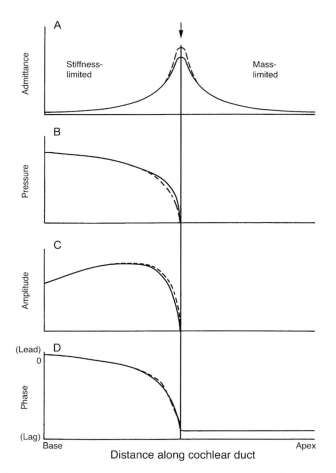

Fig. 3.15 The mechanisms giving rise to the different aspects of the broadly tuned, passive mechanical component of the travelling wave. (A) The admittance of the cochlear partition for a stimulus of one frequency is plotted as a function of distance along the cochlea. The admittance is the membrane velocity (proportional to displacement) divided by the driving pressure ratio. The admittance is highest at the resonant point (vertical line: arrow), where the effects of stiffness limitation and mass limitation cancel because they are equal in magnitude but opposite in phase. Dotted line: curve for decreased damping. (B) The pressure across the cochlear partition drops as the point of maximum admittance is reached. (C) The displacement of the cochlear partition, derived from the product of curves A and B for each point along the cochlea, shows a peak basal to the point of maximum partition admittance and a sharp drop as the point of maximum admittance is reached. (D) Phase changes along the cochlear partition.

between the base and the centre of the diagram, the admittance of the membrane increases towards the centre of the diagram, i.e. towards the apex.

Near the apical end of the cochlea, however, the admittance becomes low again because here the mass of the basilar membrane and cochlear fluids are large enough to limit the movement (see Fig. 3.15A, mass-limited right half). In between the stiffness-limited and the mass-limited portions, at the point of resonance, the effects of mass and stiffness become equal in magnitude while being exactly opposite in phase. Due to the phase opposition, their effects cancel, and the admittance becomes high. At this point, the partition therefore shows a relatively large amplitude of movement in response to a certain applied pressure difference across the partition.

For a wave that travels up the cochlear duct, we can trace the following sequence of events:

1. As the wave travels towards the apex, the admittance of the partition at first increases. The amplitude of vibration of the partition is derived from the product of the admittance and the pressure difference between the scalae, and so the wave grows in amplitude.
2. As the wave approaches the point of maximum admittance, the admittance of the partition increases still further and the amplitude of vibration increases further. However, towards the point of maximum admittance, the wave travels more and more slowly, and the effects of damping make the amplitude decline. Moreover, because of the high admittance of the membrane, the pressure difference is short-circuited across the membrane. For these reasons, the driving pressure across the membrane drops sharply as the point of maximum membrane admittance (i.e. the resonant point) is reached (see Fig. 3.15B). The amplitude of vibration, given by the product of pressure and admittance, therefore has a maximum that occurs basal to the point of maximum admittance (see Fig. 3.15C).
3. Beyond the point of maximum admittance, the movement of the partition becomes mass-limited rather than stiffness-limited. But to produce a travelling wave, we need interaction between a stiffness (in the partition) and a mass (in the fluids). Since stiffness is no longer dominant in the partition, wave motion becomes impossible. The wave therefore dies away at the point of maximum admittance, with the whole apical region of the partition moving in the same phase. The phase curve therefore becomes flat (see Fig. 3.15D).
4. Resonance occurs when stiffness and mass limitation are equal in magnitude (though opposite in phase), and this point occurs at different places along the duct, depending on the stimulus frequency. Since inertial forces are relatively greater for high-frequency stimuli, they will match the forces due to the stiffness near the relatively stiff base for high-frequency stimulation and near the apex for low-frequency stimulation. High-frequency waves therefore peak near the base of the cochlea, while low-frequency waves peak towards the apex.
5. Near the point of maximum admittance, the amplitude of the response is limited by damping, or friction, in the cochlear partition. If the damping is decreased, the peak in the admittance function becomes larger, but the travelling wave becomes only very slightly larger and only very slightly more sharply tuned (dotted lines, Fig. 3.15).

it into the marginal cells. The transporter also produces a Na^+ gradient across the junction between the marginal cells and the intrastrial fluid, which activates a $Na^+/2Cl^-/K^+$ cotransporter, further lowering the K^+ concentration in the intrastrial fluid.

K^+ diffusing from the marginal cells raises the K^+ concentration of the endolymph and also communicates the high positive potential of the intrastrial fluid and marginal cells to the endolymph. Further evidence for this model has come from demonstrations of the existence of the required channels and transporters in the required locations and from mutant mice in which different channels and transporters have been knocked out (Marcus et al., 2002; Wangemann, 2006).

Once produced, the endolymph flows out of the cochlea by way of the ductus reuniens, through the endolymphatic duct, and is absorbed in the endolymphatic sac. Malabsorption or obstruction of the flow causes an increase in the pressure of the endolymph, known as endolymphatic hydrops, such as is found in Ménière's disease (for reviews, see Paparella, 1991; Andrews, 2004).

3.3.3 The perilymph

The ionic composition of the perilymph, situated in the outer fluid compartments of the cochlea, is similar to that of extracellular fluid or cerebrospinal fluid. Its electric potential is close to that of the surrounding plasma, being reported to be +7 mV in the scala tympani and +5 mV in the scala vestibuli (Johnstone and Sellick, 1972). Perilymph appears to be at least partially produced by transcellular transport of solutes from blood plasma, likely to be via the capillaries in the walls of the perilymphatic space. In contrast to the endolymph, the perilymph has a K^+ concentration of 4–6 mM and a Na^+ concentration of 140–150 mM and is therefore similar to most other extracellular fluids (for review, see Wangemann and Schacht, 1996).

X-ray microanalysis of frozen tissue shows that the spaces within the organ of Corti have the same ionic content as perilymph (Anniko and Wroblewski, 1986). The fluid within the extracellular spaces of the organ of Corti has a potential of approximately 0 mV (Dallos et al., 1982).

3.4 HAIR CELL RESPONSES

The measurement of hair cell responses was one of the important landmarks in the progress of cochlear physiology, permitting the link to be made between the mechanical responses of the basilar membrane and the electrophysiological responses of the auditory nerve. Inner hair cells of the mammalian cochlea were first recorded from by Russell and Sellick (1978). Since the very great majority of afferent auditory nerve fibres make their synaptic contacts with inner hair cells, it must be presumed that it is the job of inner hair cells to signal the movements of the cochlear partition to the central nervous system. Outer hair cells are much more difficult to record from, and we have fewer reports. The role of the outer hair cells is to amplify the mechanical travelling wave, although the exact details of the mechanisms by which they do this are still controversial.

Hair cell responses will be dealt with in terms of the resistance–modulation and battery theory of Davis (1958), as it appears in the light of more recent evidence and summarized in Fig. 3.19. The endocochlear potential and the negative hair

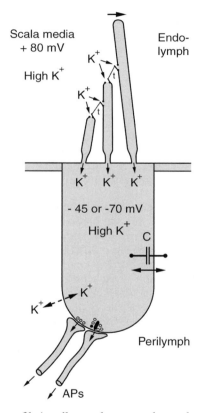

Fig. 3.19 The operation of hair cells: mechanotransducer channels at the apex of the hair cells act as variable resistances. Ions flow into the cell, driven by the battery of the endolymphatic potential and the intracellular potential. Intracellular depolarization causes the release of transmitter, and auditory nerve fibre activation. Increased current flow through the hair cells also makes the scala media less positive and the scala tympani more positive. The mechanotransducer channels (drawn here diagrammatically as little doors) are opened by tension on the tip links running between the tips of the stereocilia, as suggested by Pickles *et al.* (1984). The molecular identity of the mechanotransducer channels is not known in mammals. The large arrow shows the direction for excitatory (depolarizing) movement of the stereocilia, which is always towards the tallest stereocilia in the bundle. t: tip links. The resting potentials marked (−45 and −70 mV) are for inner and outer hair cells, respectively.

cell intracellular resting potential combine to form a potential gradient across the apical membrane of the hair cell. Movement of the cochlear partition produces deflection of the stereocilia, as shown in Fig. 3.3. Deflection in the excitatory direction (the bundle moving towards the tallest stereocilia) opens mechanosensitive ion channels in the stereocilia, by a direct mechanical action. Ions are driven into the cell by the potential gradient, causing intracellular depolarization. The depolarization causes the release of transmitter, likely to be glutamate, activating the auditory nerve fibres (see Fig. 3.19). These stages, and the evidence for them, will be dealt with in more detail in Chapter 5. Hair cell responses from non-mammalian cochleae and the vestibular system, which give basic information on the transduction process, are also dealt with in Chapter 5.

3.4.1 Hair cell responses in vitro

It is possible to isolate the cochlear sensory epithelium, namely the organ of Corti together with its surrounding structures, and mechanically stimulate the bundles of stereocilia with either a fluid jet or an applied probe. Figure 3.20 shows responses from outer hair cells recorded in such a manner. Similar responses have also been obtained from inner hair cells recorded in vitro (e.g. Russell et al., 1986a,b; Jia et al., 2007).

Movements of the hair bundle open and close the mechanotransducer channels, modulating the current through the cell. While the change in current approximately follows the waveform of the stimulus, the changes in the excitatory direction (upwards in lower part of Fig. 3.20A) are much larger than the changes in the inhibitory direction (downwards). The input–output function, which describes the moment-by-moment relation of current flow (and hence channel opening) to displacement of the hair bundle, is an asymmetric sinusoid (see Fig. 3.20B). In these particular experiments, at the resting point of the bundle (i.e. in the absence of mechanical stimulation), the channels were only slightly open, and movements in the inhibitory direction closed them completely. We can also note from Fig. 3.20B that the responses are nearly linear in the middle of the function. However, the responses also have a limited dynamic range and start to saturate for movements more than about 50 nm from the centre point of the function.

3.4.2 Inner hair cell responses in vivo
3.4.2.1 Intracellular potentials

The responses of inner hair cells can be measured in the intact cochlea, by impaling the cells with microelectrodes. The cells can then be stimulated by sounds delivered to the ear. Russell and Sellick (1978) found resting potentials of some −45 mV. This is rather more depolarized than most nerve cells, which commonly have intracellular potentials of some −70 mV.

In response to a tone of low frequency, in which the individual cycles of the waveform can be distinguished, the hair cells give potential changes which followed a distorted version of the input stimulus (upper traces, Fig. 3.21). These

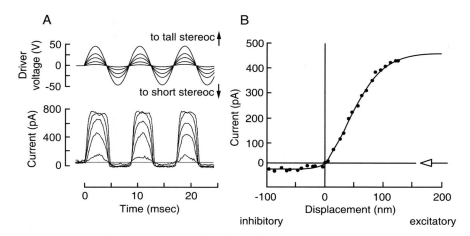

Fig. 3.20 Responses of outer hair cells recorded in vitro, in cultures from neonatal mice. In these cultures, the tectorial membrane does not develop, so hair bundles can be moved directly. The responses are recorded by a whole-cell patch-clamp electrode sealed onto the basal membrane of the hair cell. (A) Intracellular responses to sinusoidal stimulation at 100 Hz. The top trace shows the voltage applied to the driver of the fluid jet; this waveform approximates the movement of the hair bundle. The lower trace shows the current flow through the hair cell, with the cell body held at its normal resting potential via the recording electrode. The displacement of the stereocilia modulates the current through the cell, with an asymmetric response to a sinusoidal stimulus. Displacements in the excitatory direction (stereocilia moving towards the tallest in the bundle) produce much larger changes in current flow than displacements in the opposite direction (stereocilia moving towards the shortest in the bundle). From Kros et al. (1992), Fig. 3(a). (B) Responses of another cell measured in a similar manner, shown as an input–output function. During cycles of stimulation, the instantaneous displacement of the hair bundle (horizontal axis) is plotted against the instantaneous current though the cell (vertical axis). The resulting function shows the degree of channel opening as a function of displacement of the hair bundle. The horizontal line (open arrow) shows that with zero displacement of the hair bundle, the current through the cell is near zero (20 pA), i.e. the channels are only 4% open at rest. From Geleoc et al. (1997), Fig. 2(d).

responses are generally similar to those shown in Fig. 3.20, although in this case with less distortion. As with responses recorded in vitro, the excursions in the positive direction are greater than the excursions in the negative direction. It is therefore possible to describe the potential changes as an a.c. response at the stimulus frequency, superimposed on a sustained d.c. depolarization.

As the stimulus frequency is raised, the a.c. component of the voltage response declines relative to the d.c. component so that at frequencies of a few kilohertz and above, the a.c. component is much smaller than the d.c. component (lower traces, Fig. 3.21). Russell and Sellick (1983) ascribed this to the capacitance of the hair cell membranes. Hair cell membranes, like all cell membranes, have a capacitance,

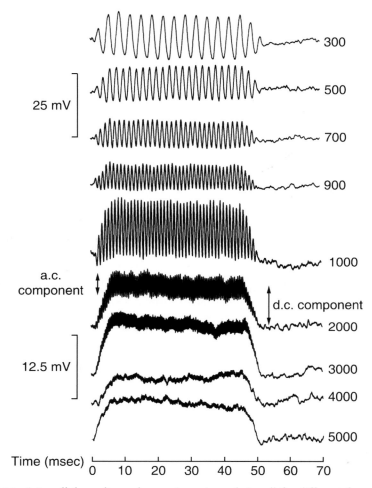

Fig. 3.21 Intracellular voltage changes in an inner hair cell for different frequencies of stimulation show that the relative size of the a.c. component declines at higher stimulus frequencies (numbers on the right of curves). Note change of scale for the lower four traces. Reprinted from Palmer and Russell (1986), Fig. 9, Copyright (1986), with permission from Elsevier.

and capacitances offer a low impedance to a.c. currents at high frequencies. At high frequencies, therefore, the a.c. current was short-circuited by the low impedance of the hair cell membranes, reducing the a.c. voltage response in the cell. Because depolarization leads to the release of transmitter at the base of the hair cells, we expect the release of transmitter, to a first approximation at least, to follow the waveforms of Fig. 3.21.

3.4.2.2 Relation to basilar membrane responses

The close correspondence between hair cell responses and basilar membrane responses can be shown in several ways. Firstly, the tuning curves for inner and outer hair cells are shown in Fig. 3.22. The curves have a low-threshold, sharply tuned tip, at the best or characteristic frequency (CF). There is also a high-threshold and broadly tuned tail, stretching to low frequencies. The shape is similar to that of the tuning curve for the mechanical response of a single point on the basilar membrane when the stimulus frequency is varied, as shown in Fig. 3.11B. The tuning of hair cells therefore appears to be derived from the tuning of the basilar membrane, although it is possible that there are some differences in the high-threshold tail.

Correspondingly, intensity functions for inner hair cells are similar to those of the basilar membrane mechanical response (Fig. 3.23A; compare with Fig. 3.13A). Around the characteristic frequency (17 kHz for this particular hair cell), the response grew linearly at first, at the rate of a 10-fold voltage change for a 20 dB increase in stimulus intensity, parallel to the dotted line. When the intensity was raised further, the response at and near characteristic frequency grew non-linearly, i.e. with a more shallow slope (remember these are log–log scales). At frequencies above characteristic frequency, the response saturated at a low maximum output voltage, while in contrast well below the characteristic frequency (e.g. 2 kHz), the response grew much more linearly. Again, both of these indicate that inner hair cell responses closely follow basilar membrane mechanical responses.

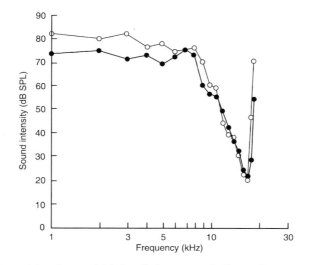

Fig. 3.22 Inner (o) and outer (•) hair cells have very similar tuning curves. The curves are also very similar to those for the mechanical response of the basilar membrane (compare to Fig. 3.11B). The IHC threshold criterion was 0.8 mV d.c. depolarization, the OHC criterion was 0.3 mV a.c. response. From Cody and Russell (1987), Fig. 7.

can show both a.c. and d.c. voltage responses. However, the voltage responses in outer hair cells are only one-half to one-third the size of those of inner hair cells, possibly reflecting the difficulty of making the recordings.

3.4.3.2 Relation to basilar membrane responses

Like inner hair cells, outer hair cells have responses that closely follow the mechanical response of the basilar membrane. Figure 3.22 shows the tuning curve for an outer hair cell a.c. response, recorded from the base of the cochlea. The frequency selectivity is very similar to that of the inner hair cell that was recorded immediately adjacent to it (Cody and Russell, 1987). Figure 3.23B shows intensity functions for the response of an outer hair cell. Again, they are generally similar to the functions of an inner hair cell (see Fig. 3.23A) and the basilar membrane (see Fig. 3.13A), although they may saturate rather more abruptly than the basilar membrane responses.

3.4.3.3 a.c. and d.c. components and input–output functions

While there is agreement about the sharpness of tuning and the general shape of the intensity functions found by the different groups of workers, there are differences in the shapes of the input–output functions and in the relative sizes of the a.c. and d.c. components of the response.

Dallos and his colleagues recorded in the apical (low-frequency) end of the guinea pig cochlea (Dallos *et al.*, 1982; Dallos, 1986). With stimulation at moderate intensities at the characteristic frequency, they showed that there was a depolarizing d.c. response superimposed on the a.c. component, in accordance with the asymmetric sinusoidal input–output function of Fig. 3.24. Unlike the position in inner hair cells, however, the function changed form as the stimulus frequency was varied, with the result that the d.c. component could become hyperpolarizing at frequencies just below characteristic frequency. If the stimulus intensity was raised, the frequency range over which depolarization could be obtained spread so that the response became consistently depolarizing.

Cody and Russell (1987), recording in the basal (high-frequency) turn of the guinea pig cochlea, found that with low-frequency stimulation, well below the characteristic frequency, the input–output function had the opposite symmetry to that shown in Fig. 3.24 – that is, the changes in the hyperpolarizing direction were greater than those in the depolarizing direction. As the stimulus frequency was raised to 2 kHz and above, the input–output functions became symmetrical so that no d.c. components were generated in the response. However, at high stimulus intensities, the response became depolarizing at all frequencies, although this happened at some 90 dB SPL, a higher intensity than in the experiments of Dallos (1986).

The differences in the input–output functions of inner and outer hair cells may be partly explained by the different ways their stereocilia are coupled to the mechanical stimulus. The stereocilia of inner hair cells are not embedded in the tectorial membrane; rather they fit loosely into the groove of Hensens's stripe and are moved by fluid flow in the subtectorial space, being driven by the velocity of the movement. Hence they are unresponsive to any static offsets or biases in the position of the basilar or tectorial membranes. In contrast, the stereocilia of outer hair cells are embedded in the tectorial membrane and will be affected by such biases. The different responses that have been measured from outer hair cells suggest that such biases or offsets in the mechanical travelling wave are a complex function of cochlear region, stimulus frequency and stimulus intensity. In particular, the lack of a d.c. response in basal hair cells to high-frequency stimulation as found by Cody and Russell (1987) suggests that under these conditions, the tectorial membrane normally biases the stereocilia to the midpoint of the input–output function of Fig. 3.20.

Russell and colleagues' high-intensity depolarizing component was rather different from the d.c. components described hitherto. Unlike the other d.c. components that appeared and disappeared instantaneously with the a.c. response, the high-intensity d.c. component in basal turn outer hair cells took several cycles to develop and several cycles to disappear after the end of the stimulus. This suggests that it cannot simply be thought of as a distortion component of the a.c. response and that a description in terms of an input–output function (see Fig. 3.20) is not appropriate. They suggested that this component of the d.c. response was due to the accumulation of K^+ ions around the basal ends of the hair cells, as a result of the acoustic stimulation.

3.5 THE GROSS EVOKED POTENTIALS

When electrodes are placed in or near the cochlea, it is possible to record gross stimulus-evoked potentials that are derived from the massed activity of large numbers of the individual receptor and nerve cells. The gross evoked potentials can be divided into three groups. Firstly, the cochlear microphonic (CM) is an a.c. response that approximately follows the acoustic stimulating waveform (Fig. 3.25). The cochlear microphonic is derived mainly from the currents flowing through the outer hair cells. Secondly, there is a d.c. shift in the record, known as the summating potential (SP), which depends on the d.c. components generated by the hair cells. Thirdly, there are a series of deflections at the beginning, and sometimes also at the end, of the stimulus, called the N_1 and N_2 neural potentials (or compound action potentials, CAP). The neural potentials are produced by the summed activity of auditory nerve fibres, producing synchronized action potentials at the onset and sometimes at the end of the stimulus.

3.5.1 The cochlear microphonic

Wever and Bray (1930) placed a wire electrode in the auditory nerve, connected to an amplifier in a room 16 m away, and from there to a loudspeaker. As they

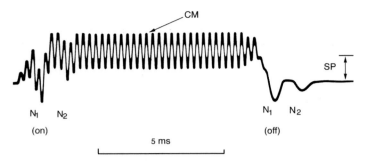

Fig. 3.25 Diagram of the response to a tone burst, recorded with gross electrodes, shows the cochlear microphonic (CM), N_1 and N_2 phases of the compound action potential (CAP) to both the beginning and the end of the stimulus and, in the d.c. shift of the microphonic from the baseline, the summating potential (SP).

reported, 'the action currents, after amplification, were audible in the receiver as sounds which, so far as the observer could determine, were identical with the original stimulus. Speech was transmitted with great fidelity. Simple sounds, commands, and the like were easily received. Indeed, under good conditions the system was employed as a means of communication between operating and sound-proof rooms.'

3.5.1.1 Generation

Tasaki *et al.* (1954) presented clear evidence as to the site of production of the cochlear microphonic. They advanced a microelectrode from the scala tympani, through the basilar membrane and the organ of Corti, into the endolymphatic space and the scala media. They recorded the cochlear microphonic as they advanced the electrode and showed that the microphonic reversed polarity at the same time as the endocochlear potential appeared. This fixes the site of generation of the cochlear microphonic as the border of the endolymphatic space, namely the reticular lamina. The reticular lamina is the surface carrying the transducing structures of the hair cells, the stereocilia. It is now clear that the cochlear microphonic is generated by the hair cells. When the transducer channels open so that current flows into the hair cells, making them more positive, current is drained from the scala media, making it less positive (see Fig. 3.19). When the channels shut, the current flow is reduced, and the scala media moves more positive. Potential changes are therefore produced, which in the scala media are in the opposite phase to the changes in the hair cells and the scala tympani.

3.5.1.2 Spatial localization

As might be expected from the mechanism of its production, the cochlear microphonic is spatially localized in the same way as the mechanical travelling wave.

Low frequencies give the greatest response near the apex and high frequencies near the base. The position of the peak of the response at low intensity compares well with the position of the peak of the travelling wave envelope (Eldredge, 1974). In addition, when the intensity is raised, the peak of the response moves towards the base of the cochlea. Part of the shift is due to the basalward shift in the travelling wave envelope at high stimulus intensities (see Fig. 3.10B).

Within the organ of Corti itself, extracellular microelectrodes situated near the basolateral walls of the outer hair cells will record the cochlear microphonic, in a form that is heavily dominated by the adjacent outer hair cells. This 'organ of Corti potential' can be used as an indicator of local outer hair cell activity and therefore can be used to draw conclusions about outer hair cell activity without the necessity of making the extremely difficult intracellular penetrations of outer hair cells (e.g. Cheatham and Dallos, 2000).

3.5.1.3 Intensity functions

With increases in intensity, responses grow similarly to those measured for the basilar membrane and outer hair cells, as shown in Figs 3.13A and 3.23B. As with the basilar membrane responses, the cochlear microphonic measured near the peak of the travelling wave grows nearly linearly only for the lowest intensities and then starts to saturate. Responses measured in the basal region of the travelling wave grow linearly with stimulus intensities to much higher intensities (e.g. to 100 dB SPL for a 1-kHz stimulus; Tasaki et al., 1952).

The cochlear microphonic can be easily recorded using an electrode placed outside the cochlea and adjacent to it. One favourite site giving good potentials is the round window, the membrane-covered opening between the scala tympani and the middle ear cavity. For low and mid-frequency stimuli, microphonics recorded from an electrode in this position, right at the base of the cochlea, will be dominated by the basal parts of the travelling wave. The round-window microphonics will therefore give an indication of the activity of the basal parts of the travelling wave and may not measure the activity produced near the peak.

3.5.2 The summating potential

The d.c. change produced in the cochlea in response to a sound is known as the summating potential (SP) and is visible as a baseline shift in the recorded signal of Fig. 3.25. Depending on the circumstances, it is recorded as a sustained positive or negative deviation in the scala media during acoustic stimulation. The summating potential has correlates in the d.c. stimulus-evoked potentials in hair cells and is probably derived directly from them. When the input–output functions of hair cells are such as to produce intracellular d.c. depolarization of the hair cells, the d.c. component of the current into the cells is greater than normal. The scala media will tend to move more negative, because of the K^+ ions moving out of the scala media, and the scala tympani will tend to move more positive. Because the intracellular d.c. depolarizations or hyperpolarizations of outer hair cells change with the stimulus parameters in a complex way (see Section 3.4.3

because it allows the auditory system to discriminate stimuli over a very wide range of stimulus intensities.

7. Deflection of the stereocilia by the travelling wave, by opening and closing ion channels in the stereocilia, modulates the current being driven into the hair cells by the combined effects of the positive endocochlear potential and the negative intracellular potential. The current produces potential changes that can be measured in the hair cells with fine microelectrodes, and grossly in the cochlea with larger electrodes.

8. Inner hair cells have resting potentials of about −45 mV. They produce both an a.c. voltage and a steady d.c. depolarization in response to sound. The potentials have sharp tuning curves and amplitude functions similar to those shown by the basilar membrane vibrations. Outer hair cells have resting potentials of about −70 mV. They show a.c. potential changes in response to sound and, depending on the circumstances, either no, or a depolarizing, or a hyperpolarizing, d.c. response. Like inner hair cells, they show sharp tuning curves and amplitude functions similar to those shown by basilar membrane vibrations.

9. The potential changes in inner hair cells serve to govern the release of neuro-transmitter, probably glutamate, to produce action potentials in the auditory nerve fibres. Outer hair cells amplify the mechanical travelling wave, pro-ducing a mechanical motile response in the hair cells. The motile response may arise from one or both of the following: (1) a lengthwise contraction and expansion of the outer hair cell body in response to intracellular depo-larization and hyperpolarization or (2) Ca^{2+} ions entering though the open mechanotransducer channels, which may change the conformation of the mechanotransducer apparatus, leading to an output of mechanical energy that can feed back into the mechanical system.

10. The cochlear microphonic is the extracellular correlate of the a.c. current flowing through hair cells. It is generated predominantly by outer hair cells. The summating potential is primarily the extracellular correlate of the d.c. component of the current flowing through hair cells. Depending on circum-stances, it can be recorded as either a positive or a negative shift in the scala media and probably receives contributions from both inner and outer hair cells, and possibly from other sources.

11. The massed synchronized activity of auditory nerve fibres, called the compound action potential (CAP) or the N_1 and N_2 potentials, can be recorded with gross electrodes in response to stimulus onsets.

3.7 FURTHER READING

Cochlear anatomy has been reviewed by Santi and Mancini (2005) and cochlear anatomy and biology by Raphael and Altschuler (2003). Differences in cochlear anatomy between animals and human beings have been reviewed by Felix (2002). The molecular anatomy of the mechanotransducer apparatus has been reviewed by Vollrath *et al.* (2007). Molecular aspects of cochlear physiology in relation to pathology have been reviewed by McGee and Walsh (2005). Cochlear mechanics have been reviewed by Robles and Ruggero (2001), and by Patuzzi (1996), de Boer (1996) and Ricci (2003). The electrochemical environment of the cochlea has been reviewed by Wangemann and Schacht (1996) and Wangemann (2006). Hair cell responses have been reviewed by Kros (1996) and the role of prestin in cochlear amplification by Dallos *et al.* (2006). Mechanisms of transduction are further dealt with in Chapter 5 of the present work.

CHAPTER FOUR

THE AUDITORY NERVE

We now have a comprehensive description of the responses of auditory nerve fibres to a variety of stimuli in normal, albeit anaesthetized, animals. We also understand some of the changes that occur in auditory nerve activity during cochlear pathology. The responses of auditory nerve fibres underlie the responses of the later stages of the auditory system and closely relate to the psychophysical capabilities of the intact organism. For these reasons, knowledge of the material presented in this chapter is essential for the understanding of the later chapters on the central auditory system (Chapters 6–8), psychophysical correlates of auditory physiology (Chapter 9) and sensorineural hearing loss (Chapter 10). Those whose later interest is primarily in Chapter 10 need here only read up to and including Section 4.2.2.

4.1 ANATOMY

Auditory nerve fibres, with their cell bodies in the spiral ganglion, provide a direct synaptic connection between the hair cells of the cochlea and the cochlear nucleus. Each ear has about 50 000 fibres in cats and 30 000 in human beings (Harrison and Howe, 1974a, Felix, 2002). The very great majority (90–95%, depending on species) of auditory nerve fibres make their synaptic contacts directly and exclusively with the inner hair cells (Spoendlin, 1972; Liberman et al., 1990). A diagram summarizing Spoendlin's scheme is shown in Fig. 3.6. The reader is reminded that the fibres innervating the inner hair cells innervate the hair cells nearest to their point of entry into the cochlea, whereas those innervating the outer hair cells run basally for about 0.6 mm before terminating. About 20 afferent fibres innervate each inner hair cell (Fig. 4.1), whereas about 6 fibres innervate each outer hair cell. Each fibre to the inner hair cells connects with one and only one hair cell, whereas those to the outer hair cells branch and innervate about 10 hair cells (Simmons and Liberman, 1988). Differentiation in the targets is associated with a morphological differentiation in the cell bodies and axons. A total of 95% of cells (in cats) connect with the inner hair cells, have bipolar cell bodies in the spiral ganglion, and have myelinated cell bodies and axons (Spoendlin, 1978). They are

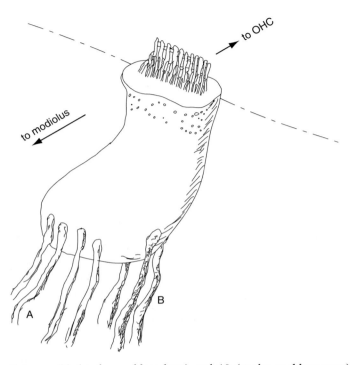

Fig. 4.1 Between 30 (at the cochlear base) and 10 (at the cochlear apex) Type I afferent auditory nerve fibres (radial fibres) make contact with each inner hair cell. The fibres (A) contacting the hair cell on the modiolar side of the cell have smaller diameters, higher thresholds in response to acoustic stimulation, and low rates of spontaneous firing. The fibres (B) on the outer hair cell side or tunnel side of the inner hair cell have larger diameters, low thresholds, and high rates of spontaneous firing. This diagram shows only 7 of the 30 synapses expected on a basal inner hair cell. Data from Tsuji and Liberman (1997).

called Type I cells. Type II cells connect with outer hair cells, are monopolar, and are not myelinated. Retrograde transport of horseradish peroxidase from the cochlear nucleus to the cochlea confirms that both types send axons to the cochlear nucleus (Ruggero *et al.*, 1982).

It is generally thought that the very great majority of auditory nerve responses have been measured from Type I cells. Type I cells are typically driven strongly by tones and can show high levels of spontaneous activity. We have only one confirmed instance, by tracing a horseradish peroxidase injection, of a record from a Type II cell (Robertson, 1984; see also Robertson *et al.*, 1999). Here, the cell was silent in response to acoustic stimulation. We do not therefore know the function of the Type II system in audition, although some ideas will be discussed in Chapter 5.

4.2 PHYSIOLOGY

We must assume, provisionally at least, that all, or substantially all, the auditory nerve fibres or cells that have been recorded from innervate the inner hair cells. Although our knowledge of the responses of inner hair cells is still relatively sketchy, we do have a fairly complete knowledge of the responses of the auditory nerve. Our knowledge has accumulated over the past 40 years or so and has depended on a careful control of stimulus and physiological parameters, together with the surveying of large populations of fibres, sometimes as many as 418 fibres in one animal (Kim *et al.*, 1980). This has been achieved in spite of the inaccessibility of the nerve deep in the bone, and the lack of mechanical stability of the adjacent brainstem, which means that nerve fibres can easily be lost in recording. In fact, it was not until 1954 that the first responses of auditory nerve fibres were published (Tasaki, 1954), and it is now recognized that the records indicate that the cochlea must have been in poor physiological condition. Tasaki's approach was to drill through the temporal bone until the auditory nerve was encountered in the internal auditory meatus. The approach commonly used nowadays is to open the occipital bone at the back of the skull and, by inserting a retractor around the edge of the cerebellum, to retract the cerebellum and the brainstem medially away from the wall of the skull until the stub of the nerve running between the internal auditory meatus and the cochlear nucleus becomes visible. Microelectrodes can then be inserted under direct vision. Alternative approaches are to record from cells of the spiral ganglion directly through holes in the cochlear wall or to record from within the internal auditory meatus by means of microelectrodes inserted stereotaxically through the brainstem. When appropriate measures are taken to stabilize the preparation, fibres or cells can now be recorded for many tens of minutes, compared to the 10 s or so managed by Tasaki.

With microelectrodes with a tip size 0.3 μm or less, single fibres can be recorded from and give waveforms corresponding to those in Fig. 4.2. Many fibres

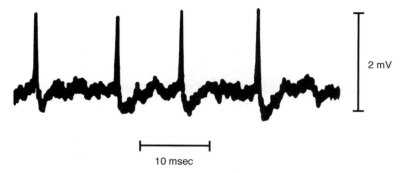

2 mV

10 msec

Fig. 4.2 Action potentials recorded extracellularly from a single auditory nerve fibre. The waves are initially positive and nearly monophasic. Photograph by courtesy of G. Leng.

show random spontaneous activity. There is a bimodal distribution of spontaneous discharge rates. About a quarter of the fibres discharge at below 20/sec, and most of these discharge at 0.5/sec or less. The other group has a mean of 60–80 discharges/sec, with a maximum of 120/sec (Evans, 1972; Liberman and Kiang, 1978).

4.2.1 Response to tones

4.2.1.1 Threshold responses and frequency selectivity

Fibres are responsive to single tones, and in the absence of other stimuli the tones are always excitatory and never inhibitory. The responses can be demonstrated by means of a post- (or peri-) stimulus–time histogram (post-stimulus-time histogram). In making such a histogram, a stimulus is presented many times, and the occurrence of each action potential is plotted on the histogram by incrementing the count on the column, or bin, corresponding to the time after the beginning of the stimulus. Tone bursts produce a sharp onset response, which drops rapidly over the first 10–20 ms (Fig. 4.3), and then more and more slowly over the next several minutes. The fibres can be characterized by their threshold as a function of frequency of the tone. The intensity of a tone burst is adjusted until an increment in firing is just detectable. This increment is commonly between 5 and 30 spikes/sec, depending on the spontaneous firing rate of the fibre and the method used to detect the increment. The procedure is repeated for different frequencies of stimulation. Examples of the resulting tuning curves relating threshold to frequency are shown in Fig. 4.4. Each fibre has a low threshold at one frequency, the 'characteristic'

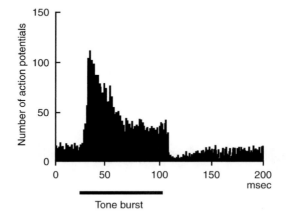

Fig. 4.3 Single fibres of the auditory nerve show an initial burst of activity at the beginning of a tone burst, a gradual decline, and a transient off-suppression of the spontaneous activity at the end of the stimulus. Here, a post-stimulus-time histogram was made by presenting tone bursts many times and incrementing the count at the corresponding point on the histogram whenever an action potential occurred. Author's data.

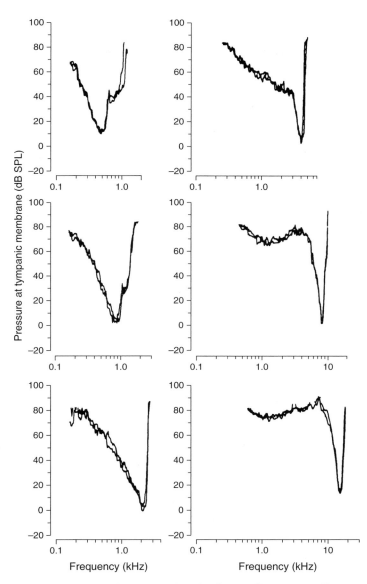

Fig. 4.4 Representative tuning curves (FTC) of cat auditory nerve fibres are shown for six different frequency regions. In each panel, two fibres from the same animal of similar characteristic frequency and threshold are shown, indicating the constancy of tuning under such circumstances. Reprinted from Liberman and Kiang (1978), Fig. 1, with permission of Taylor and Francis Ltd (http://www.informaworld.com).

or 'best' frequency, and the threshold rises rapidly as the stimulating frequency is changed.

Figure 4.4 shows the typical change in shape of tuning curves across frequencies, if the frequency scale is logarithmic. At low frequencies, below 1 kHz, tuning curves are nearly symmetric. At higher frequencies, the curves become increasingly asymmetric, with steep high-frequency slopes and less steep low-frequency slopes. A distinction between two parts of the tuning curve also becomes obvious in high-frequency units. There is a very sensitive, frequency-selective 'tip' of the tuning curve and a long, broadly tuned 'tail', stretching to low frequencies. The tail has a broad dip around 1 kHz. This is probably derived from the boost given to the input by the middle ear characteristics, since it disappears if the stimulus intensity is plotted with respect to constant stapes velocity (Kiang et al., 1967). Single auditory nerve fibres therefore appear to behave as band-pass filters, with an asymmetric filter shape. The frequency selectivity is similar to that of the basilar membrane and the hair cells, from which their frequency selectivity is derived (see Figs 3.11B and 3.22; Ruggero et al., 1997).

All mammals investigated show tuning curves broadly similar to those of Fig. 4.4, although details such as the degree of frequency selectivity and the depth of the tip may vary from species to species.

Liberman (1978) showed that there is a 60–80 dB spread of fibre thresholds at any one characteristic frequency. Ninety percent of fibres have high spontaneous firing rates and have thresholds within the bottom 10 dB of the range. The remainder, which have medium and low spontaneous rates, are spread over the rest of the range (Fig. 4.5).

Intracellular labelling of nerve fibres after electrophysiological recording shows that fibres with different thresholds and spontaneous rates can innervate the same inner hair cell. The differences must therefore be due to differences in the fibres or synapses, rather than to differences in the hair cells themselves (Tsuji and Liberman, 1997). In addition, there are anatomical variations in the fibres with different physiological properties. Fibres with high levels of spontaneous activity are thicker than the others and innervate the pillar (i.e. non-modiolar or outer hair cell) side of the inner hair cells, while fibres with low and medium rates of spontaneous activity are finer and innervate the modiolar side (Liberman, 1982; Tsuji and Liberman, 1997).

The degree of frequency selectivity has been expressed in two ways. One is by the slopes of the tuning curve above and below the characteristic frequency. The slopes are a function of the characteristic frequency of the fibres concerned, with, in many species, the fibres in the 10-kHz region having the steepest slopes. Here the high-frequency slopes measured between 5 and 25 dB above the best threshold range from 100 to 600 dB/octave, and the low-frequency slopes from 80 to 250 dB/octave (Evans, 1975). Further up the slope of the tuning curves, the low-frequency slopes become shallower as the 'tail' is approached, but the high-frequency slopes become even steeper, sometimes increasing to as much as 1000 dB/octave (Evans, 1972).

A second way that resolution can be expressed is by measuring the bandwidth of the tuning curve at some fixed intensity above the best threshold. By analogy

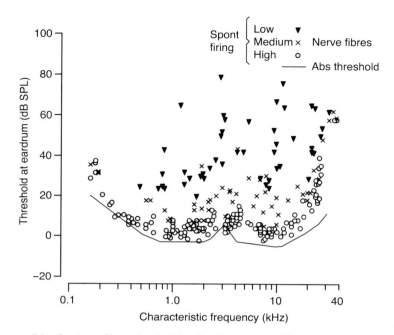

Fig. 4.5 Distribution of best thresholds of auditory nerve fibres in a cat. Fibres with high spontaneous firing rates (○, ≥18 per second) have low thresholds, and those with low spontaneous firing rates (▼, <0.5 per second) have high thresholds. Fibres with intermediate spontaneous firing rates (×) have thresholds in between. The behavioural absolute threshold of the cat, expressed in terms of the intensity at the eardrum, lies just below the lowest thresholds of the auditory nerve fibres. Neural data reprinted from Liberman and Kiang (1978), Fig. 2. Behavioural data from Elliott *et al.* (1960), with permission of Taylor and Francis Ltd (http://www.informaworld.com).

with the practice in the measurement of the bandwidths of electrical filters, it might be thought appropriate to measure the half-power bandwidth, i.e. the bandwidth 3 dB above the best threshold. However, because it is difficult to measure thresholds sufficiently accurately, bandwidths 10 dB above the best threshold have been used instead. The 10-dB bandwidths plotted as a function of characteristic frequency show a restricted spread (Fig. 4.6A). A related way in which the resolution can be expressed is by analogy with the electrical 'quality' or 'Q' factor of a filter, defined as the centre frequency divided by the bandwidth, the bandwidth here being defined at 10 dB above the best threshold. The quality factor so defined is called Q_{10} or $Q_{10\,dB}$, and a high-quality factor, or high Q_{10}, corresponds to a narrow bandwidth. Figure 4.6B shows that for cats the minimum relative bandwidth occurs around 10 kHz, where it averages about one-eighth of the characteristic frequency. Comparable values have been measured for basilar membrane and hair cell responses (Russell and Sellick, 1978; Sellick *et al.*, 1982; Ruggero *et al.*, 1997; see also Robles and Ruggero, 2001 for review).

averaging techniques some phase-locked responses are detectable up to 12 kHz (Recio-Spinoso et al., 2005).

Phase locking is a sensitive indicator of the activation of a fibre by a low-frequency tone. At low stimulus intensities, a tone can produce significant phase locking even though the mean firing rate is not increased. Tuning curves based on a criterion of a certain degree of phase locking are similar to those based on an increase in firing rate, although for the above reason they may be more sensitive by 20 dB or so (Evans, 1975). As the intensity is raised, phase locking is preserved (see Fig. 4.9). Note that, although the total number of spikes evoked does not increase above 70 dB SPL, meaning that the firing rate is saturated, the period histogram still follows the waveform of the stimulus and does not show any sign of squaring. This occurs because the hair cells' a.c. responses are still approximately sinusoidal at high stimulus intensities (Dallos, 1985).

4.2.2 Response to clicks

A click, which lasts a short time but which spreads spectral energy over a wide frequency range, can be thought of as the spectral complement of a tone, which lasts a long time but which has only a narrow frequency spread. Figure. 4.10 shows the

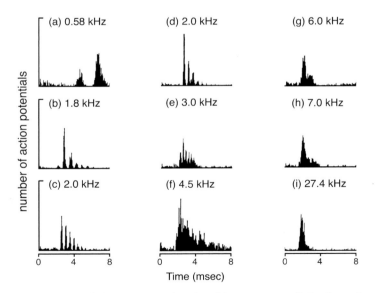

Fig. 4.10 The form of the post-stimulus-time histograms to clicks depends on the characteristic frequency of the fibre. Low-frequency fibres show ringing (a–e) at the characteristic frequency, whereas high-frequency fibres do not (f–i). High-frequency fibres also show a later phase of activation (g), corresponding to a response to the broad dip seen in the tail of the tuning curve of high-frequency fibres (Fig. 4.4). From Kiang et al. (1962), Fig. 5.

post-stimulus-time histograms of the auditory nerve fibres to clicks. The histograms of low-frequency fibres show several decaying peaks. It looks as though they would be produced by a decaying oscillation, i.e. as though the basilar membrane rings in response to the stimulus. The frequency of the ringing is equal to the characteristic frequency of the cell (Kiang *et al.*, 1965). This ringing at the characteristic frequency is exactly what would be expected if the tuning of the auditory nerve fibres was produced by an approximately linear filter. We would also expect the rate of decay of the ringing to be inversely proportional to the bandwidth of the tuning curve, so that a sharply tuned fibre would ring for a long time.

As with the response to tones, it appears as though only one phase of the basilar membrane movement is effective. The histogram corresponds to half cycles of the decaying oscillation produced on the basilar membrane (Fig. 4.11A). As with tones, for low-frequency fibres it appears as though the velocity of movement of the membrane towards the scala vestibuli is responsible for excitation, since for these fibres at high stimulus intensities, a rarefaction click produces the earliest activation (see Fig. 4.11B). An approximate picture of the excitatory oscillation can be produced by inverting the histogram of a condensation click under that of a rarefaction click, to produce what has been called a compound histogram (see Fig. 4.11C). Histograms to clicks can also show that the suppression of activity during the less effective half cycle of the stimulating waveform is not due to refractoriness from previous activity, because the first sign of influence on a fibre can sometimes be a suppression of spontaneous activity produced by the less effective half cycle.

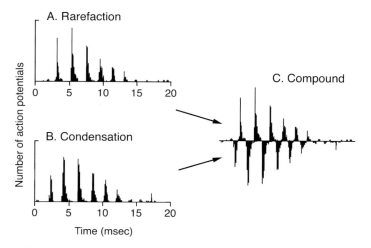

Fig. 4.11 (A) Post-stimulus–time histograms to (A) rarefaction and (B) condensation clicks show that the peaks and troughs occur in complementary places for the two stimuli. (C) A compound histogram is formed by inverting the histogram of condensation clicks under that of rarefaction clicks. Reprinted from Goblick and Pfeiffer (1969), Fig. 1, Copyright (1969), with permission from American Institute of Physics.

4.2.4 Response to complex stimuli

4.2.4.1 Two-tone suppression

It was stated above that single tones produce excitation in auditory nerve fibres, and never sustained inhibition. However, the presence of one stimulus can affect the responsiveness of nerve fibres to other stimuli, and if the relative frequencies and intensities of two tones are arranged correctly, the second tone can inhibit, or suppress, the response to the first. This can occur even though the second tone produces no inhibition of spontaneous activity when presented alone. Figure 4.13 shows the post-stimulus-time histogram produced by a suppressing tone superimposed on a continuous excitatory tone. The pattern of response to the suppressing tone looks like the inverse of the pattern to an excitatory one. The suppressing tone produces an initial maximum of suppression when turned on and produces a prominent rebound of activity when turned off. The dip in activity at the beginning of the suppressing tone looks like the transient suppression seen at the end of an excitatory stimulus, and the activity at the end looks like the onset burst seen at the beginning of an excitatory stimulus (cf. Fig. 4.3). This suggests that the suppressing tone simply turns the effect of the excitatory tone off. The fact that only stimulus-evoked, and not spontaneous, activity can be suppressed makes the same point.

Arthur *et al.* (1971) made detailed measurements of the relative latencies of excitation and suppression to tone onsets and found that on average excitation

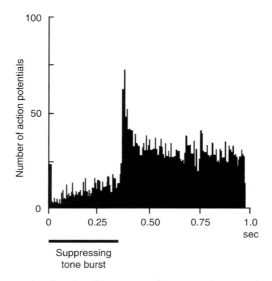

Fig. 4.13   The post-stimulus–time histogram of a suppressing tone burst superimposed on a continuous excitatory tone. Reprinted from Sachs and Kiang (1968), Fig. 1, Copyright (1968), with permission from American Institute of Physics.

and suppression differed in latency only by 0.1 ms. The latency of suppression has more recently been measured by measuring the temporal fluctuations in the response to one tone, when a low-frequency suppressing tone is superimposed (e.g. van der Heijden and Joris, 2005). These results suggested that, when travel times along the cochlear duct were taken into account, suppression occurs on a time-scale of about two cycles. The very short time constants of suppression suggest very strongly that suppression is not the result of inhibitory synapses in the cochlea, even if possible synapses had been demonstrated anatomically, because there is no time for synaptic delay (about 1 ms). The latency argument also means that the suppression cannot be a result of the activity of the olivocochlear bundle, the 'feedback' pathway from the brainstem nuclei to the hair cells (see Chapter 8), as has also been confirmed by direct experiment (Kiang et al., 1965). Because it is believed that two-tone suppression is not the result of inhibitory synapses, the more neutral term 'suppression' rather than 'inhibition' is often used. Of course, 'inhibition' is still used for the process mediated by inhibitory synapses, which is seen in the later stages of the auditory system, in, for instance, the cochlear nucleus. 'Suppression' is used only for the process occurring in the cochlea.

It is now clear that suppression occurs at the mechanical stage. Two-tone suppression can be seen in the vibration of the basilar membrane, and in the responses of cochlear hair cells (Sellick and Russell, 1979; Ruggero et al., 1992). The basilar membrane and the hair cells have the advantage over the auditory nerve in that it is easier to assess the effects of the exciting and suppressing tones separately. In the case of the hair cell shown in Fig. 4.14, the excitatory tuning curve was first assessed from the d.c. response to an excitatory tone. The cell was then stimulated with a continuous tone (the probe), having the intensity and frequency indicated by the triangle in Fig. 4.14. A suppressive tone was then swept across the response area, and the contours for 20% suppression of the a.c. response at the probe's frequency determined (Sellick and Russell, 1979). The results show that the suppressing tone can reduce the response to the exciting tone when presented over a wide range of frequencies. The suppressive area is more broadly tuned than the excitatory response area and overlaps it at the tip. In other words, a stimulus can suppress even though it does not excite and can still suppress the response to another stimulus, even though it excites when presented alone.

The overlap of excitatory and suppressive areas that has been demonstrated in inner hair cells can also be shown in auditory nerve fibres, for tones of low frequencies, by taking advantage of the fact that the firing will follow the waveform of an exciting stimulus. If two tones are presented, the firing will follow the waveform of the sum of the two in an appropriate combination of amplitude and phase. By looking at the degree of phase locking of the firing to any one tone in a complex, it is possible to calculate the degree to which the fibre is activated by that frequency component and to measure the extent to which the response to that component is suppressed by the other stimulus. In this way, Javel et al. (1983) showed that the narrow excitatory response area was overlaid by a broader suppressive area.

If, of course, the second tone is in the suppressive area but outside the excitatory area, it will be easy to measure the suppression by measuring the total firing

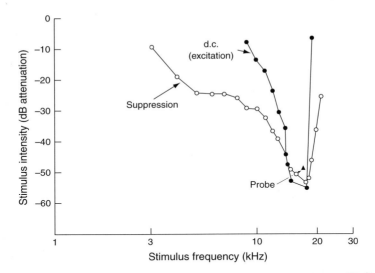

Fig. 4.14 Excitatory and suppressive tuning contours for an inner hair cell. The d.c. contour is the d.c. depolarization to a single tone and shows the excitatory tuning curve. The triangle shows the frequency and intensity of the probe tone, and the open circles show the contour for 20% suppression of the a.c. response to the probe. All stimuli within the excitatory contour excite, and all within the suppressive contour suppress. Stimuli within both contours both suppress and excite. Reprinted from Sellick and Russell (1979), Fig. 3, Copyright (1979), with permission from Elsevier.

rate to the stimulus complex. The second tone produces only suppression and does not contribute any excitation of its own. The overall mean firing rate will then be a measure of the activation produced by the excitatory tone and the extent to which it is suppressed by the suppressor. Plots of the combinations of intensity and frequency necessary to reduce the mean firing rate in response to a constant excitatory tone by a certain criterion amount (20% has been commonly taken) show the suppressive areas where they flank the excitatory area (Sachs and Kiang, 1968; Arthur *et al.*, 1971; Fig. 4.15A). When the suppressing tone reaches the boundary of the excitatory area, it will begin to activate the fibre on its own account, and so the total number of action potentials will increase. Suppression areas plotted in this way therefore stop at, or near, the boundary of the excitatory area.

It is most likely that two-tone suppression derives from the non-linear responses of outer hair cells as shown in the saturating input–output function of Fig. 3.20B. When hair cells are stimulated with one stimulus, a superimposed stimulus will drive the stereocilia to greater displacements, i.e. further into the flatter part of the input–output curve. Because of the non-linearity of the outer hair cells' responses, the response in the outer cells to the two stimuli together will be less than the sum of the responses to the two stimuli considered separately. Therefore, each stimulus will reduce the active amplification of the travelling wave

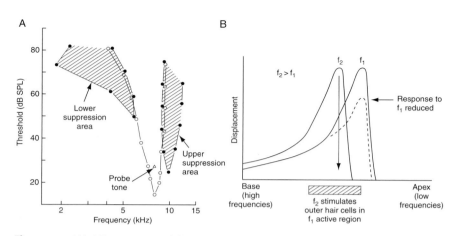

Fig. 4.15 (A) The upper and lower suppression areas of an auditory nerve fibre (shaded) flank the excitatory tuning curve (open circles). A stimulus in the suppression areas was able to reduce the mean firing rate found with the probe by 20% or more. From Arthur *et al.* (1971), Fig. 2. (B) Two-tone suppression explained where the suppressor (f_2) is of higher frequency than the suppressed tone (f_1). The travelling wave to the higher-frequency tone overlaps the region on the basilar membrane where the travelling wave to the lower-frequency tone is being actively amplified. Because of the saturating non-linearity in the responses of outer hair cells, this reduces the active amplification produced by the lower-frequency tone. This explanation holds where the excitatory areas of the suppressor and suppressed tones overlap, and in the upper suppression area of part (A).

to the other one. (In addition, of course, the non-linearity means that each stimulus could be said to reduce the active amplification of its own travelling wave, resulting in the saturating non-linearity of basilar membrane intensity functions.)

This explains two–tone suppression where both tones are in the excitatory part of the tuning curve, such that their travelling waves overlap. Similarly, we can see how a higher-frequency tone might be able to suppress, even though it does not excite (e.g. in the upper shaded two–tone suppression area of Fig. 4.15A). As shown in Fig. 4.15B, a higher-frequency suppressor produces a travelling wave on the basilar membrane, with a peak basal to that produced by the exciter, or probe, tone. This will overlap the region where the active amplification of the suppressed tone f_1 is occurring, and so reduce the amplification of f_1. Further up the cochlea, the travelling wave to the high-frequency suppressor f_2 will be filtered out by the mechanics, leaving the wave to the lower-frequency tone f_1, but at a reduced amplitude (Fig. 4.15B).

Note, however, that this explanation of how a stimulus can suppress without causing excitation does not apply to the low-frequency suppression area. The mechanism of low-frequency two–tone suppression is at the moment controversial and will be discussed further in Chapter 5.

Suppression has a number of effects of the discriminability of auditory stimuli, depending on circumstances. Figure 4.15A indicates that a stimulus is able to reduce the driven response of fibres tuned to neighbouring frequencies. Two-tone suppression is therefore potentially able to increase the contrast in a complex sensory pattern, so that, for instance, the peaks of activation produced by dominating frequencies will tend to stand out in stronger contrast against the background. However, because suppression reduces the active mechanical amplification in the cochlea, it makes the cochlea more linear, less sensitive, and more broadly tuned, which will tend to reduce resolution. The possible effects of two-tone suppression on the discrimination of complex stimuli will be discussed in Chapter 9.

4.2.4.2 Masking

Masking denotes the general phenomenon in which one stimulus obscures or reduces the response to another. We can identify three mechanisms of masking:

1. *The 'line busy' effect.* If one stimulus has pre-empted the firing of a fibre, superimposed stimuli will not be able to provoke an increment in firing. In one statement of the hypothesis, if the firing is saturated to one stimulus, superimposed stimuli will not be able to increase the rate further (Smith, 1979). This mechanism will also be operative to some extent below saturation. If one signal has a greater effective intensity than the other, the less intense one will add negligible activity of its own. Such an effect will be greater than might appear at first sight, because the summation of effective intensities will occur on a linear scale rather than on the logarithmic scale of decibels. For instance, a signal added 10 dB below another will produce an increase in net stimulus intensity of only 0.4 dB.
2. Two-tone suppression, by the mechanism discussed above, reduces responses and broadens tuning to the suppressed stimulus (Pang and Guinan, 1997b).
3. Adaptation forms a further mechanism of masking: in response to prolonged background stimulation, the firing rate that can be evoked by a transient superimposed stimulus is reduced, presumably due to depletion of neurotransmitter at the hair cell synapse.

Figure 4.16 shows an example of masking by all three mechanisms. The figure shows rate-intensity functions for a tone both with and without wideband masking noise. The tone alone could produce a maximum firing rate just over 300/sec. The continuous noise was then presented at an intensity that gave a firing rate of 160/sec. Tones were superimposed on the noise; tones less intense than 50 dB SPL did not produce a greater firing rate than the noise, and so did not increase the response. In this intensity range, the tone was masked by the line busy effect. Once the tone is intense enough to activate the fibre in the presence of the noise, its rate-intensity function in noise is seen to be shifted 10 dB to the shifted 10 dB to the right compared with that without noise, showing the effects of suppression. In addition, for the most intense tones, the maximum firing rate to the tone plus

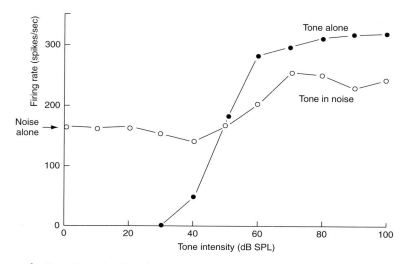

Fig. 4.16 Rate–intensity functions to a tone with and without masking noise. The tone was presented at 2.9 kHz, the CF. The noise band was centred around the CF and covered 2.5–4 kHz. At low tone intensities, the noise activates the fibre on its own ('line busy' effect). At higher tone intensities, it is possible to see how the noise reduces the response to the tone. Suppression by the noise also shifts the tone's rate–intensity function to the right. Used with permission from Rhode *et al.* (1978), Fig. 3E.

noise is lower than to the tone alone. This shows the effect of both adoptation and suppression.

   We are now in a position to understand some of the complex interactions between the components of multicomponent stimuli. If two stimuli of comparable levels are presented, both well inside the excitatory area, each will suppress the other strongly, but both will excite the fibre even more strongly. Below saturation, the firing rate in response to both will be greater than that to either one alone, and they will therefore appear to summate in their effects. For low-frequency units, the firing will follow a waveform that can be composed of the waveforms of the component stimuli added together with suitable amplitudes and phases (Rose *et al.*, 1971). The relative amplitudes and phases giving the best fit are not necessarily those presented in the acoustic stimulus. The frequency selectivity of the fibre, as well as the mutual suppression of the components, will alter their relative amplitudes. In the case of the phases, the effects of suppression are complex and not entirely understood (see Chapter 5).

   In a more trivial case where one stimulus has much less influence over the fibre than the other, the most effective stimulus will dominate both the firing rate and the temporal pattern of the action potentials. When the effects of suppression are strong, the temporal pattern can follow the waveform of the suppressing as well as of the exciting stimulus (Rose *et al.*, 1971).

4.3 SUMMARY

1. The very great majority of the fibres present in the auditory nerve innervate inner hair cells.
2. Single fibres of the auditory nerve are always excited by auditory stimuli and never show sustained inhibition to single stimuli.
3. The fibres have lower thresholds to tones of some frequencies than of others. The relation between threshold and stimulus frequency is known as the 'tuning curve'. Turning curves show one threshold minimum, at what is known as the characteristic frequency. The threshold rises sharply for frequencies above and below the characteristic frequency. The tuning curve therefore shows a sharp dip in this frequency region. Tuning curves of auditory nerve fibres are similar to the tuning curves of hair cells and of the mechanical response of the basilar membrane.
4. The great majority (90%) of auditory nerve fibres have minimum thresholds in a 10-dB range near the animal's absolute threshold. The others have thresholds spread over a 60-dB range above that. The low-threshold fibres have particularly high rates of spontaneous activity in the absence of sound.
5. Fibres show a sigmoidal relation between firing rate and stimulus intensity. Low-threshold fibres also have steeper rate-intensity functions, often going from threshold to maximum rate in 20–30 dB (the dynamic range) at any one frequency. Fibres of higher threshold have shallower rate-intensity functions and wider dynamic ranges, up to 60 dB or more.
6. The frequency-resolving power of auditory nerve fibres has been measured by a 'quality' factor, by analogy with a quality factor for filters. The quality factor is the characteristic frequency divided by the bandwidth of the fibre to tones at an intensity 10 dB above the best threshold. This is called 'Q_{10}' or 'Q_{10dB}'. Therefore, fibres with a high Q_{10} have good frequency selectivity. At any one frequency, different fibres have Q_{10}s in a restricted range. In any one animal, the range of Q_{10}s at one frequency is two-fold or less. In cats, the greatest Q_{10}s are reached at around 10 kHz, where they have an average value of eight. The Q_{10}s match, to a first approximation at least, the Q_{10} of the basilar membrane vibration.
7. During tonal stimulation, auditory nerve fibres fire preferentially during one part of the cycle of the stimulating waveform if the stimulus is below 4–5 kHz. The fibres are excited by deflection of the basilar membrane in only one direction.
8. For fibres with characteristic frequencies below 4–5 kHz, clicks preferentially evoke responses at certain intervals after the stimulus. A histogram of action potentials made with respect to time after the stimulus suggests that the fibres are activated by the half cycles of a decaying oscillation of the mechanical resonance on the basilar membrane. The frequency of the oscillation is equal to the characteristic frequency of the fibre.
9. One tone can reduce, or suppress, the response to another, even though single tones are only excitatory. This is called two-tone suppression. The suppression

arises from the non-linear properties of the basilar membrane mechanics. Two-tone suppression can also be seen in the basilar membrane mechanics and the responses of inner hair cells. Stimuli other than tones cause suppression too.

10. One stimulus can mask the response to another. Masking mainly occurs because the masking stimulus produces a greater firing rate than the masked stimulus. The other mechanisms of masking are the suppression of the response to one stimulus by another, and adaptation in the fibre produced by an ongoing stimulus.

11. When two-tone stimuli are used, auditory nerve fibres can respond to distortion products as a result of non-linear interactions in the cochlea. One distortion tone, known as the cubic distortion tone, is at a frequency $2f_1 - f_2$, where f_1 is the lower of the tones presented and f_2 the higher.

4.4 FURTHER READING

The auditory nerve has been reviewed by Ruggero (1992). Some information is also included in a review of cochlear mechanics by Robles and Ruggero (2001).

mechanotransducer channels are dependent on the mechanical properties of the stereocilia and the way in which the stereocilia are coupled together. In response to deflection of the stereocilia, a shear is developed between the different rows of stereocilia on the hair cell, which is then coupled to fine tip links, of macro-molecular dimensions, which transmit the movement to the transducer channels themselves.

In addition, outer hair cells are known to be motile and actively gener-ate movements when stimulated. The exact mechanism behind the motility is uncertain: the motility may depend on reverse motion generated by the mechan-otransducer channels in the apical portions of the hair cells, or on a specialized motor protein, called prestin, in the basal membranes of the cells. This motility is responsible for amplifying the mechanical travelling wave on the basilar membrane and for generating the sharply tuned, low-threshold component of the mechanical response.

5.2 THE STRUCTURE OF THE TRANSDUCER REGION

5.2.1 Stereocilia and cuticular plate

Micromanipulation experiments show that stereocilia act as stiff, rigid, levers, bending only at the point of insertion into the cuticular plate and fracturing as though brittle when pushed too far (Flock *et al.*, 1977). Stereocilia gain their considerable rigidity from a core of tightly packed actin filaments. The actin fil-aments are tightly bonded together in what is known as a paracrystalline array, the high degree of bonding contributing to the rigidity to the stereocilia (Tilney *et al.*, 1980). After acoustic overstimulation, the paracrystal is seen to be disor-dered, with an irregular spacing of the filaments in longitudinal view and loss of the striations due to bonding (Tilney *et al.*, 1982). The regions of disorder are associated with a bending or kinking of the stereocilia. This suggests that the mechanical rigidity of the stereocilia is indeed associated with the integrity of the paracrystal.

Within the paracrystal, all the actin filaments have the same polarity so that when decorated with the heavy (S1) fragments of myosin, the S1 fragments make a pattern of arrowheads pointing down into the cell body (Tilney *et al.*, 1980; Fig. 5.1). This also has the implication that actin–myosin interactions in living cells will tend to carry the myosin molecules up towards the tips of the stereocilia. The actin filaments are cross-linked by means of the actin-linking proteins fimbrin and the espins, shown by means of immunological techniques. A mutation in the espin gene in the strain of mice known as jerker mice leads to stereociliar degeneration, deafness and vestibular dysfunction, and a similar changes have been detected in human beings (Zheng *et al.*, 2000b; Donaudy *et al.*, 2006). The tip region of the stereocilia is capped by different myosins (3a and 15a), each with a different distribution (Schneider *et al.*, 2006).

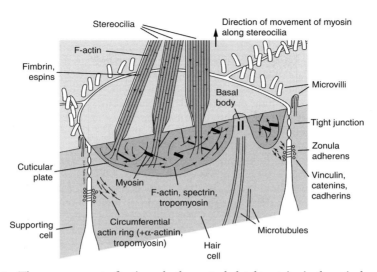

Fig. 5.1 The arrangement of actin and other cytoskeletal proteins in the apical regions of hair cells. The molecular organization of the upper ends of the stereocilia is shown separately in Fig. 5.7. Arrows show the direction of the arrowhead complexes formed after decoration with myosin heads (S1-myosin), and show the similarity of stereocilia to microvilli. The links between the actin filaments are also shown. From Pickles (2007b).

The stereocilium is able to flex at its lower end, just before it enters the cuticular plate, because it tapers at this point before continuing into the cuticular plate as a dense rootlet. About 10 (counted in the lizard basilar papilla) of the actin filaments in the stereocilium enter the rootlet in this way, the rest ending in association with the membrane of the stereocilium where it tapers (Tilney *et al.*, 1980).

The cuticular plate itself is also composed of actin filaments, here in a dense meshwork. The cuticular plate also contains tropomyosin, α-actinin (a component of the muscle Z-line), myosin, fimbrin, profilin, tropomyosin and the Ca^{2+} binding proteins calbindin and calmodulin (for review, see Slepecky, 1996). It has been suggested that spectrin, originally known as a component of the erythrocyte membrane, bonds the matrix of the cuticular plate to the overlying membrane (Drenckhahn *et al.*, 1985). The dense matrix of interlinked actin filaments in the cuticular plate would be expected to give the plate considerable rigidity.

In contrast to the apparently haphazard matrix of filaments in the cuticular plate, organized actin filaments can be found running in a ring-like arrangement just inside the zonula adherens at the apical end of the hair cell. The rings contain actin filaments oriented in opposite polarities. The suggested arrangements of actin filaments and associated cytoskeletal structures in the apical region of hair cells are shown in Fig. 5.1.

5.2.2 The cross-linking of stereocilia

The stereocilia in a hair bundle are heavily cross-linked in a variety of ways. The stereocilia are bonded together sideways by links that run predominantly parallel to the cuticular plate. The side links run between the stereocilia of the different rows on the hair cell as well as between the stereocilia of the same row (Pickles *et al.*, 1984). These side links probably serve to couple the stereocilia mechanically, with the result that in micromanipulation experiments all stereocilia in a bundle tend to move together when some are pushed. Figure 5.2 shows an example of the side links running between stereocilia of the same row on an inner hair cell, and Fig. 5.3 shows side links joining stereocilia of different rows. The side links (arrowheads, Fig. 5.3) are concentrated in a broad band just below the tips of the shorter stereocilia and hold the tips of the shorter stereocilia near the adjacent taller stereocilia. The rows of stereocilia therefore make triangles when seen in sideways view.

The links of a second set are rather different and have generated interest because they couple the stimulus-induced movements to the transducer areas of the stereocilia (Pickles *et al.*, 1984). A single vertically pointing link emerges from the tip of each shorter stereocilium on a hair cell and runs up to join the adjacent taller stereocilium of the next row. The links are 130–200 nm long. Figure 5.3 shows these tip links by transmission electron microscopy and Fig. 5.4A by scanning electron microscopy. Each tip link consists of a fine 8–11-nm strand, surrounded by a variable coat (Osborne *et al.*, 1988; Gillespie *et al.*, 2005). Figure 5.4B and C shows the central strand in more detail. It bifurcates at the top end and at

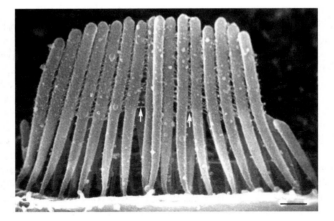

Fig. 5.2 Inner hair cell of the guinea pig cochlea, showing side links (arrows) running between the stereocilia of the tallest row on the hair cell. Note also that the surface membranes of the stereocilia appear rough, particularly at the level of the links. Scale bar, 500 nm.

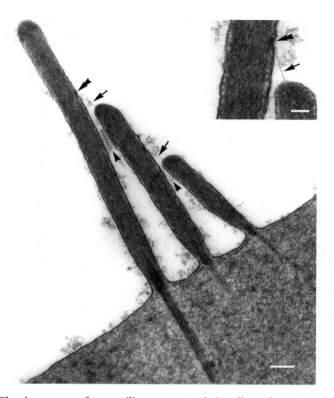

Fig. 5.3   The three rows of stereocilia on an outer hair cell are shown in cross section. The stereocilia of the different rows are joined by horizontal (between-row) side links just below their tips (arrowheads). The inset shows a higher magnification of the lower tip link. Tip links (arrows) have a fine central core, surrounded by amorphous material (see also inset). Double arrowhead: upper density. Guinea pig. Scale bar on main figure: 200 nm, on inset 100 nm. Reprinted from Osborne *et al.* (1988), Figs 3 and 4, Copyright (1988), with permission from Elsevier.

high resolution has a spiral structure (Kachar *et al.*, 2000; Tsuprun *et al.*, 2004). The link inserts into specialized densities in the stereocilia, while the surrounding coat is probably a continuation of the glycoconjugate material that surrounds the surfaces of the stereocilia (Santi and Anderson, 1987). As suggested by Pickles *et al.* (1984), if the tallest stereocilium in Fig. 5.3 were deflected away from the shorter stereocilia, the tip links would tend to be stretched. This could pull open mechanotransducer channels situated at the links' points of insertion into the stereocilia, by a direct mechanical action (Fig. 5.5).

The physical nature of the link is important because the link has to be able to transmit very small (subnanometre) displacements to the transducer channel,

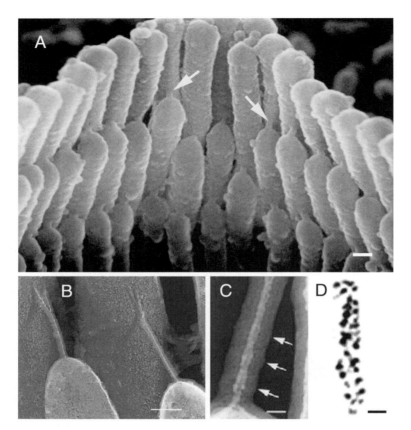

Fig. 5.4 (A) Tip links (arrows) shown by scanning electron microscopy, in the apex of the 'V' of stereocilia on a guinea pig outer hair cell. The stereocilia were photographed nearly parallel to the axis of bilateral symmetry, showing that the tip links run parallel to that axis, i.e. parallel to the excitatory–inhibitory axis, and approximately radially across the cochlear duct. In this micrograph, the central cores of the tip links are covered by glycocalyx. Scale bar, 200 nm. (B) The central cores of two tip links shown at higher resolution, by freeze-etch transmission electron microscopy, and showing how the links bifurcate at their upper ends. The preparations were frozen and fractured, the surface was given texture by permitting evaporation, and then was coated with platinum and carbon to give a layer that could be visualized with a transmission electron microscope. Scale bar, 100 nm. From Kachar *et al.* (2000), Fig. 3A, Copyright (2000), National Academy of Sciences, USA. (C) A tip link at higher magnification, prepared with the same technique, showing the spiral structure. Arrows point to repeats of the spiral. Scale bar, 15 nm. From Kachar *et al.* (2000), Fig. 2C, Copyright (2000), National Academy of Sciences, USA. (D) The fine structure of a part of a tip link, obtained from a noise-filtered electron micrograph image at high magnification. Globular elements are visible aligned in two spiral strands. Scale bar, 10 nm. From Tsuprun *et al.* (2004), Fig. 1E.

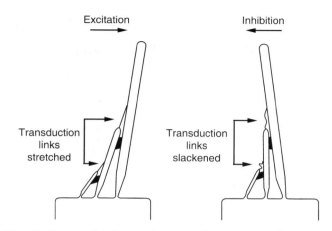

Fig. 5.5 The tip link model for mechanotransduction, according to Pickles *et al.* (1984). Deflection of the bundle in the direction of the tallest stereocilia, which is always the excitatory direction, applies tension to the links and pulls open the mechanotransducer channels. Deflection in the reverse direction takes tension off the links and allows the channels to close. Reprinted from Pickles *et al.* (1984), Fig. 9, Copyright (1984), with permission from Elsevier.

while being able to accommodate the very large – micron – extensions that occur when the bundle undergoes large deflections. There is considerable evidence that a cell adhesion molecule, cadherin-23, is a component of the tip link. Sollner *et al.* (2004) looked for auditory and vestibular dysfunction in populations of randomly mutated zebrafish. They found one line of fish, called 'sputnik' because the fish swam in circles, where the dysfunction was associated with mutations of the gene encoding cadherin-23. In these fish, the tip links were absent. At the same time, in mouse and bullfrog hair cells, Siemens *et al.* (2004) showed antibody labelling to cadherin-23 on or near the tip links. In human beings, defects in the cadherin-23 gene lead to hearing loss in one type of the Usher syndrome (reviewed by Petit, 2001). However, whether the extracellular strand of the tip link is composed only or principally of cadherin-23 and the associated protein protocadherin-15 is at the moment not known (Gillespie *et al.*, 2005; Kazmierczak *et al.*, 2007).

In addition to electrophysiological evidence to be described in the next section, supporting anatomical evidence for the role of tip links in mechanotransduction are the following:

(1) Their position on the stereocilia, being ideal to detect excitatory movements of the bundle (see Fig. 5.5).

(2) They are the only structures known that are oppositely stressed by excitatory and inhibitory deflections of the stereocilia, through the different types of manipulations (e.g. pushing or pulling the bundle) that have been used experimentally.

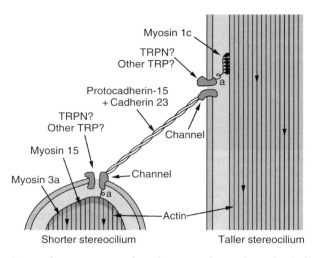

Fig. 5.7 Conjectured arrangement of mechanotransducer channels, tip link and associated proteins are shown for a tip link between a taller and a shorter stereocilium (e.g. as in inset to Fig. 5.3). Where the identification is still not entirely certain, a query is shown. The mechanotransducer channels are shown situated in the membrane at either end of the tip link. The tip link, of which components are probably cadherin-23 and protocadherin-15, is here drawn as inserting directly onto the channel, although it may connect via an intermediary protein and may itself insert directly into the membrane. The channel is provisionally shown as being tethered to the underlying cytoskeleton via (in the case of zebrafish TRPN) its ankyrin repeats (a), which may act as the gating spring (see kinetic analysis of mechanotransduction). A group of myosin 1c molecules at the upper end of the tip link forms an intermediary between the channel and the underlying actin filaments; the myosin heads tend to crawl up the actin filaments, tensioning the tip link as part of the slow adaptation mechanism. Myosin 3a and 15a form parts of the cap over the actin filaments at the tips of stereocilia. Other proteins (e.g. the actin-bundling protein espin and harmonin, which can associate with cadherin-23) are known in the region, but are not shown here. Arrows on actin filaments show the direction of arrowheads formed by decoration of actin by myosin heads. Myosin tends to actively move along the actin filaments in the opposite direction to the arrows. Data from Pickles *et al.* (1984, 1991), Dumont *et al.* (2002), Sidi *et al.* (2003), Corey (2006), Rzadzinska *et al.* (2004, 2005), Siemens *et al.* (2004), Schneider *et al.* (2006) and Vollrath *et al.* (2007) and Kazmierczak *et al.* (2007).

5.3 THE ELECTROPHYSIOLOGICAL ANALYSIS OF TRANSDUCTION

It is difficult to record intracellularly from single cochlear hair cells while manipulating the stereocilia, and so the best information on transduction has been obtained from hair cells of the vestibular system. However, where data from cochlear hair cells are available, they have supported the data from vestibular cells.

Before considering the process of transduction, it is useful to review a few of the basic facts about cell membrane potentials.

5.3.1 Cell membrane potentials

Nerve cell membranes are more permeable to some ions than to others – for instance, in the resting state they are many more times permeable to K^+ than to Na^+ ions. Because there is a high K^+ concentration inside the cell and because the cell membrane is permeable to K^+, K^+ ions tend to diffuse out passively down their concentration gradient, taking positive charge with them and leaving the inside of the cell with a net negative potential. This potential is known as a diffusion potential. Diffusion continues until the negative potential inside the cell is sufficient to stop further movement of ions, at which point in an ideal system K^+ would be held in equilibrium. The value of potential at which this occurs is known as the equilibrium potential. It is possible to think of various schemes for the modulation of ion flows in hair cells. If, for instance, the apical surface of the hair cell faced an endolymph that, as well as having a low electrical potential, had a low K^+ concentration, increasing the permeability to K^+ alone would generate a negative diffusion potential across the apical membrane of the hair cell. K^+ would tend to diffuse out of the hair cell, tending to take the membrane towards the K^+ equilibrium potential. The inside of the cell would then become hyperpolarized, i.e. more negative. Increasing membrane permeability alone does not therefore necessarily produce a reduction in the membrane potential; the important point is that the membrane potential tends to move in a direction towards the equilibrium potential of the diffusible ion, or to a weighted mean of the various equilibrium potentials if more than one ion is involved.

In mammals the K^+ concentration in endolymph is approximately the same as that inside the cell, and the Na^+ concentration is very low. Therefore no substantial diffusion potential will be produced by the flow of these ions across the apical membrane of the hair cell, and decreasing the resistance will simply pull the intracellular potential towards the endolymphatic potential, producing a depolarization. As a bonus, in mammals the endolymphatic potential is 80 mV or so positive. This increases the driving force across the apical membrane from 45 mV or so to 125 mV in the case of the inner hair cells.

It is presumably advantageous for the current to be carried by K^+ rather than by Na^+. Because K^+ is in equilibrium across the basal membrane of the hair cell, any K^+ entering the cell will diffuse out automatically through K^+ channels in the basal membrane, and K^+ will not accumulate inside the cell. In this case, the energy driving the current flow is ultimately derived from ion pumps in the stria vascularis. It has the advantage of allowing the main blood supply to be removed well away from the organ of Corti, with a consequent reduction in possible vascular noise.

Although there are considerable advantages in the transducer current being carried by K^+, we must not forget that other schemes are possible. For instance, if the apical surface faced a normal extracellular fluid that was high in Na^+ and externally applied stretch of the gating spring, the energy difference ΔG between the closed and open states becomes $\kappa xy + C$.

From Boltzmann's law, the probability p_1 that a system at equilibrium is in state 1 rather than the probability p_2 that it is in state 2 is related to the energy difference ΔG between the states, according to the following formula:

$$p_1/p_2 = e^{-\Delta G/kT}$$

where k is the Boltzmann's constant and T the absolute temperature.

Here

$$p_c/p_o = e^{-\Delta G/kT},$$

where $p_o = p(\text{open})$ and $p_c = p(\text{closed})$. Because at equilibrium $p_o + p_c = 1$,

$$p_o = \frac{p_o}{p_o + p_c} = \frac{1}{1 + (p_c/p_o)} = \frac{1}{1 + e^{-\Delta G/kT}} = \frac{1}{1 + e^{-(\kappa xy + C)/kT}}$$

This is the basic formula that relates the open probability of the channel at equilibrium to the extension of the gating spring x produced by an external stimulus, in the two-state kinetic model. Because the stretch of the gating spring can be related to the deflection of the stereociliary bundle by simple geometry, the open probability can now be related to the deflection of the bundle. The function is a symmetrical sigmoid, going from zero open probability at large negative deflections to open probability of one at large positive deflections. This function corresponds to the relation between open probability and magnitude of the input stimulus for some (e.g. Fig. 5.13), but not all (see, e.g., Fig. 3.20B) experimental results. Apart from the position of the curve along the horizontal axis, the only free parameter that needs to be adjusted in fitting the theoretical function is the product κy, which is equal to the effective stiffness of the gating spring multiplied by the swing of the channel's gate; in the case of Fig. 5.13, this had a value of 4.3×10^{-14} N per channel.

Where experimental functions deviate from the symmetric sigmoid, the function commonly saturates relatively sharply for low open probabilities and saturates relatively slowly for high open probabilities (as in Fig. 3.20B). This can be accounted for with a model with three or more states, by supposing that, as with many other channels, there are at least two closed states C_1 and C_2 and one open state (see, e.g., Corey and Hudspeth, 1983; Markin and Hudspeth, 1995).

The model explains some otherwise curious results, such as the way in which the time constants of channel opening decrease for large stimulus steps (Corey and Hudspeth, 1983). This occurs because the energy of the closed state (upper curve, Fig. 5.12B) becomes larger with larger deflections of the stereocilia so that the energy barrier for opening defined in Fig. 5.12B becomes smaller relative to the closed state, with the result that the transitions become faster. In addition, it suggests that the channel does not have any absolute threshold for opening, since the opening is probabilistic, under the influence of thermal energy. Such processes are required to account for the very low threshold of auditory sensitivity.

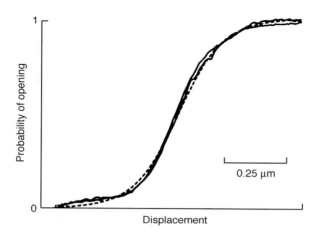

Fig. 5.13 Symmetrical change in transducer current, as recorded with a patch–clamp electrode in a single cell of the bullfrog sacculus. The curves for the measured transducer current (solid lines) have been fitted with a curve calculated from the two-state kinetic model described in the text (dotted line). From Holton and Hudspeth (1986), Fig. 12.

The energy diagram of Fig. 5.12B has another implication. As an external force moves the channel from its closed state to the open state, the channel has to move over the energy barrier between the states. Once just over the top of the barrier, the channel will tend to jump spontaneously to the next energy minimum, the open state. From the top of the barrier, therefore, the gate will move spontaneously in the direction of the applied force, or in other words, show a negative stiffness. This can be detected as a drop in the stiffness of the bundle as a whole (Howard and Hudspeth, 1988; Markin and Hudspeth, 1995). The fact that channel opening and closing can affect the stiffness of the whole bundle is a strong confirmation of the idea that the channels are opened by a direct mechanical action.

The anatomical structure that corresponds to the gating spring is at the moment uncertain. Initially it was suggested that the tip link was elastic and that the link, as well as coupling the mechanical stimulus to the mechanotransducer channel, could act as the gating spring. However, the micrographs of Kachar *et al.* (2000) suggested that the link might be stiff, not elastic, and if the link is composed of cadherin-23, it is difficult to see how cadherin-23 could have sufficient elasticity. Instead, attention has more recently been focussed on proteins that have many ankyrin repeats like TRPN1 or ankyrin itself. Molecular modelling of the behaviour of the repeats suggests that they should act as an elastic spring, of approximately the same elasticity and extensibility as the gating spring (Sotomayor *et al.*, 2005). If this were the case, Fig. 5.12 would have to be revised, with the gate being opened by a relatively rigid link (the tip link), and the channel as a whole being attached to the underlying cytoskeleton by the elastic gating spring, formed by the ankyrin repeats. However, the basic kinetic analysis of the gating spring model would remain unchanged.

5.3.2.7 Adaptation

When hair cells are stimulated with a sustained deflection of the stereocilia, their responses decline over time (Fig. 5.14A). In cochlear hair cells, the adaptation occurs with a time constant of 0.15–4 ms. This adaptation, known as fast adaptation, has been seen in hair cells of the turtle cochlea as well as the mammalian cochlea (Kros *et al.*, 1992; Ricci *et al.*, 2000; Kennedy *et al.*, 2003; see also review by Fettiplace, 2006). Fast adaptation can be affected by manipulations that alter the Ca^{2+} levels within the stereocilia, such as varying the external Ca^{2+} concentration

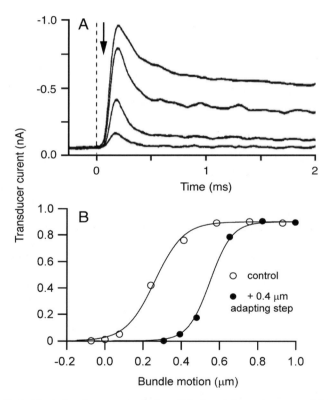

Fig. 5.14 Fast adaptation in an outer hair cell isolated from the rat cochlea. (A) The responses to steady displacement steps applied to the stereocilia decline with time. For the second smallest step in (A), the time constant was 0.16 ms. The arrow shows the moment at which the deflection of the bundle started. Reprinted from Kennedy *et al.* (2003), Fig. 1, Copyright (2003), with permission from Macmillan Publishers Ltd: Nature Neuroscience. (B) Response of an outer hair cell of the rat cochlea as a function of displacement of the stereocilia, before (control) and nearly immediately (5 ms) after an adapting step. From Fettiplace (2006), Fig. 1B.

(since Ca^{2+} enters through the mechanotransducer channels), depolarizing the hair cells to prevent Ca^{2+} from entering, or experimentally varying the intracellular concentration of Ca^{2+} buffers such as BAPTA (Ricci et al., 1998). The rapid action of Ca^{2+} that enters through the mechanotransducer suggests that it acts within 15–35 nm of the channel. On a current model, the Ca^{2+} binds within the mechanotransducer channel, making it more likely to close. This shifts the channel's operating point so that the channel requires a larger stimulus force to open, lowering the open probability (Fig. 5.14B; Wu et al., 1999; Cheung and Corey, 2006). The shift in the operating point actively adjusts the point on the input–output function at which the cells remain when there is no applied displacement to the stereocilia (see, e.g., Fig. 3.20B). When adapted, the cells do not lose overall responsiveness, because the slope of the activation curve remains steep. The time constant of fast adaptation varies with cochlear location, being faster in hair cells tuned to high frequencies (Ricci et al., 2005).

Vestibular hair cells and turtle cochlear hair cells also show another type of adaptation, called slow adaptation, which occurs over a longer timescale of 20 ms or more. Slow adaptation, like fast adaptation, causes a shift in the operating point of the hair cell along the displacement axis. However, unlike fast adaptation, which probably depends on a change in the gating properties of the mechanotransducer channel, slow adaptation depends on a geometrical change within the stereociliary bundle. The polarity of the actin filaments of the stereocilia, as shown by the arrowheads formed when the filaments are decorated with heavy actin heads (S1 myosin), suggests that the myosin 1c at the upper end of the tip link would tend to crawl up the actin filaments within the stereocilia, towards the tips of the stereocilia, thereby tensioning the tip link and pulling the mechanotransducer channels open (see Fig. 5.7). The entry of Ca^{2+} though open mechanotransducer channels tends to make the myosin motor slip so that the adaptation mechanism comes to equilibrium when the entry of Ca^{2+} through the partially open channels is just sufficient to hold the motor back against the tension of the tip link and the channels, thus setting the zero point of the bundle. Slow adaptation, unlike fast adaptation, can be affected by intracellular myosin ATPase inhibitors (see Gillespie, 2004 for review). It is possible that slow adaptation does not exist in mammalian cochlear hair cells, because it has not been seen in electrophysiological records. However, the candidate myosin, myosin 1c, is expressed at the requisite sites on the hair cell stereocilia (Dumont et al., 2002).

5.4 THE ORIGIN OF SHARP TUNING IN THE COCHLEA

As described in Chapter 3, passive mechanical models of the cochlea have difficulty in reproducing the low-threshold, sharply tuned component of the travelling wave. The only theories to be successful in matching mechanical, hair cell, and auditory nerve tuning suppose that the cochlea contains an active mechanical amplifier. The amplifier, probably involving the outer hair cells, detects the movement of the basilar membrane and feeds mechanical energy back into the

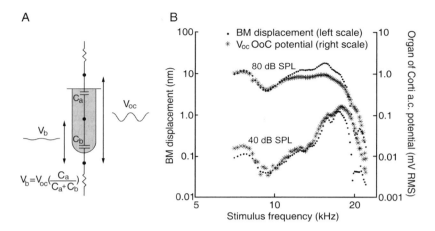

Fig. 5.21 (A) According to the suggestion of Dallos and Evans (1995a,b), at high frequencies, when most of the transcellular currents pass through the capacitances of the outer hair cell membranes, the apical and basal capacitances of an outer hair cell (shown in A) will act as a simple voltage divider. Mechanotransducer currents produce an oscillating voltage across the organ of Corti (V_{oc}). Since the impedance of a capacitor C is proportional to $1/C$, the voltage across the basal membrane of adjacent hair cells $V_b = V_{oc}\, C_a/(C_a + C_b)$. The estimated values of C_a and C_b suggest that V_b should be about 20% of V_{oc}, with the ratio being substantially independent of frequency above about 2 kHz. C_a and C_b are the capacitances of the apical and basal membranes of the hair cell. (B) High-frequency extracellular voltages within the organ of Corti are detectable and nearly proportional to basilar membrane displacement as a function of frequency. Figure supplied by Dr. A. Fridberger (original data from Fridberger *et al.*, 2004).

5.4.5.2 Motility of hair cell stereocilia

Motility of different types has been seen in stereociliar bundles of hair cells of different types and from different species. Stereociliar-based motility is moreover the only option in non-mammalian species and mammalian vestibular hair cells that do not have the basal membrane specializations of mammalian outer hair cells. For instance, Martin *et al.* (2003) showed that hair cells of the bullfrog sacculus could sometimes spontaneously oscillate at frequencies between 5 and 50 Hz. The oscillation was affected by manipulations that would affect the myosin slow adaptation motor (Section 5.3.2.7) and was therefore thought to depend on the activity of the myosin molecules found at the upper ends of the tip links (see Fig. 5.7). Any myosin-based motility would, however, be too slow to serve motility in cochlear hair cells in the auditory range of frequencies. Any such motility is instead thought to depend on rapid Ca^{2+}-induced conformation changes within the mechanotransducer apparatus (Cheung and Corey, 2006). Different forms of fast stereocilia-based motility have been observed; in rat cochlear outer hair cells, Kennedy *et al.* (2005, 2006) found that the stereociliar bundles could produce an active movement to a stimulus that was in the same direction as the applied force. This could potentially magnify the movement to the stimulus. In contrast, in the turtle cochlea, stimulation generated a delayed movement opposite in direction to the applied force (Ricci et al., 2000). Both types of motility were accompanied by a Ca^{2+}-dependent closure of the channels. It therefore appears that both types of motility may be related to fast adaptation, although with different mechanisms in the two cases, because the opposite effects were produced on bundle movement. For the type seen in the rat outer hair cell, one can speculate that the conformational change is an expansion of a protein situated between the channel and the gating spring or the tip link; this moves the bundle further in the excitatory direction, while shutting the channel. For the type seen in the turtle cochlea, one can speculate that Ca^{2+} forces the channel to shut without altering the geometry of its connections so that closure of the channel would pull the bundle in the inhibitory direction. The second type of motility is probably responsible for the stimulus-triggered active oscillations of the stereociliar bundle that can be seen in turtle cochlear hair cells (Crawford and Fettiplace, 1985). Either type of motility could generate a power stroke, if Ca^{2+} altered the conformation of a protein in a concentration-dependent manner, since Ca^{2+} ions are driven into the hair cell by the electrochemical gradient across its apical surface. Hair bundle motility, and its possible relation to channel adaptation, have been reviewed by Fettiplace (2006).

5.4.5.3 Conclusions on hair cell motility

Outer hair cell somatic motility definitely exists; the transmembrane voltages may go to sufficiently high frequencies to drive the motility in many mammalian species, although this is still uncertain particularly for very high-frequency mammals such as bats. Also uncertain is how the somatic motility is coupled to drive the vibrations of the basilar membrane. Stereocilia-based motility, probably dependent on a conformational change in the mechanotransducer apparatus, has been demonstrated in non-mammalian hair cells and in isolated mammalian cochlear hair cells, but it is still not certain whether it amplifies vibrations in the intact cochlea. It is possible that both types of motility contribute together to the amplification of the travelling wave. Neither type of motility intrinsically incorporates a mechanism to confine the active process to the rising region of the travelling wave.

5.5 HAIR CELLS AND NEURAL EXCITATION

5.5.1 Stimulus coupling to inner and outer hair cells

The tips of the tallest stereocilia of outer hair cells are embedded in the tectorial membrane, while the stereocilia of inner hair cells fit loosely into a groove called Hensen's stripe without any evidence that the tips are embedded. This has suggested that, while the stereocilia of outer hair cells are moved directly by displacements of the tectorial membrane, the stereocilia of inner hair cells are moved by viscous drag of the fluid in the subtectorial space. Since viscous drag is dependent on the velocity of the flow, we would expect that for low frequencies of stimulation, inner hair cells would respond to the velocity of basilar membrane movement, while outer hair cells would respond directly to the displacement.

Dallos *et al.* (1972) and later Sellick and Russell (1980) stimulated the cochlea with a low-frequency triangular acoustic wave, which is calculated to give a trapezoidal pattern of displacement on the basilar membrane. They showed that the above conjecture was indeed the case, with inner hair cells giving a large response in phase with the velocity of the movement, and with the cochlear microphonic, generated by the outer hair cells, following the displacement (Fig. 5.22). In accordance with the functional polarization of hair cells, depolarization in inner hair cells was produced by velocity towards the scala vestibuli, which can be expected to displace the stereocilia in the excitatory direction, i.e. in the direction of the tallest stereocilia (see Figs 3.3 and 3.19). Such a velocity response can, however, only be expected for low frequencies of stimulation; above about 1 kHz, the viscous drag becomes strong enough to convert the inner hair cell response to a displacement response (Patuzzi and Yates, 1987). The low-frequency velocity coupling of the inner hair cells suggests that they would not be directly sensitive to any d.c. bias in the position of the basilar membrane, but would only pick up the a.c. component in the vibration. On the other hand, outer hair cells would be directly affected by d.c. biases in the position of the membrane, and this may be important in affecting

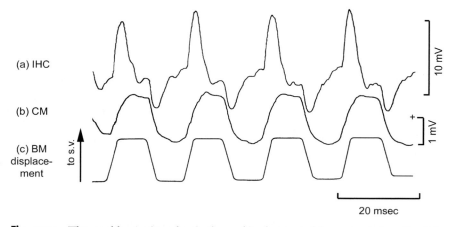

Fig. 5.22 The cochlear microphonic (trace b), dominated by outer hair cells, follows the displacement of the basilar membrane (trace c), whereas the inner hair cell responses (trace a) follow the velocity. In both cases, movement towards the scala vestibuli caused positivity below the reticular lamina, indicating a similar functional polarization for inner hair cell and outer hair cells. In this figure, recordings were made from the base of the guinea pig cochlea. The velocity response has also been confirmed for inner hair cells from the apex of the cochlea (Cheatham and Dallos, 1999). The displacement of the basilar membrane was calculated from the rate of change of sound pressure applied to the ear. Reprinted from Sellick and Russell (1980), Fig. 1, Copyright (1980), with permission from Elsevier.

the way they produce the hypothesized active mechanical feedback. The two types of coupling can therefore be associated with the different roles of the two types of hair cells in cochlear function, with inner hair cells detecting the movement of the membrane and the outer hair cells helping to generate it.

5.5.2 Activation of auditory nerve fibres

The phase of activation of the auditory nerve afferents by the inner hair cells is a complex issue and one that has not been fully resolved. On the basis of the above analysis, we would expect auditory nerve fibres to be activated in phase with the velocity of the basilar membrane movement towards the scala vestibuli, since this is the phase giving inner hair cell depolarization. This is indeed the case for fibres innervating the apical regions of the cochlea (Ruggero and Rich, 1987; Cheatham and Dallos, 1999).

The position is different, however, for the base of the cochlea. As expected, peak inner hair cell responses occur in phase with the maximum velocity of the basilar membrane movement towards the scala vestibuli, as shown in Fig. 5.22. However with low intensity stimuli, auditory nerve fibres in this region have a response phase that is nearly 180° different from the expected value, corresponding instead most closely to the maximum velocity towards the scala tympani (Fig. 5.23A). This of course could be determined only at low frequencies, in the frequency range for phase locking of the auditory nerve fibres. Figure 5.23A also shows that as the intensity is raised, at about 85 dB SPL, there is an abrupt jump in the phase of activation of the auditory nerve fibres so that at that intensity and above, the peak phase of activation now most closely corresponds to the peak velocity to the scala vestibuli, in agreement with the direction initially expected. Similar jumps in the phase of activation of auditory nerve fibres have been known for many years (e.g. Kiang and Moxon, 1972). Figure 5.23B shows how the rate-intensity function can also suddenly dip at this point. In the region of the dip, the period histogram becomes more complex, with multiple phases of activation, while the phase reverses on either side of the dip (see Fig. 5.23C). A reasonable hypothesis to explain the results is that there are two modes of activation of the auditory nerve fibres, one associated with high intensities of stimulation, and the other with low, and that they are in phase opposition. At some intensity in between, the two modes can cancel, giving rise to a dip in the response and the abrupt phase shift. At this point, small differences between the waveforms of the two driving stimuli become apparent in the period histogram.

Because of the phase of the auditory nerve responses at high stimulus intensities, depolarization of the inner hair cells is likely to form the high–intensity mode of activation. The second process must therefore drive the activation at low intensities. One candidate for the low-level excitation is the a.c. extracellular current flowing through the outer hair cells, which can be sufficient to reverse the expected a.c. voltage change across the inner hair cell synapses (Cheatham and Dallos, 1999). The result is that displacement of the basilar membrane towards the scala tympani, which causes hyperpolarization of the outer hair cells and of the spaces of the organ of Corti, can drive the release of neurotransmitter at

probably depends on changes in Ca^{2+} levels further away from sites of Ca^{2+} entry, and which is likely to involve the release of vesicles that are stored further away in the cell. This phase is likely to permit continued firing during long acoustic stimuli and to support the spontaneous activity of the nerve fibre.

Auditory nerve fibres differ in spontaneous activity and threshold, fibres with high levels of spontaneous activity having lower thresholds (see Fig. 4.5). All nerve fibres innervate the same population of inner hair cells, and it is easy to see how threshold and spontaneous activity could be dependent on the same mechanism, with low-threshold fibres having lower thresholds for release of neurotransmitter. However, we have no further information on the origin of the difference or the relative contributions of presynaptic and postsynaptic mechanisms (see, e.g., Merchan-Perez and Liberman, 1996).

5.6 COCHLEAR NONLINEARITY

One of the most intriguing aspects of cochlear function is its nonlinearity. The nonlinearity of the basilar membrane vibration is produced by the process generating sharp tuning. That process, namely the active amplification of the travelling wave by the outer hair cells, derives most or all of its nonlinearity from the intrinsic nonlinearity of hair cell transduction. Cochlear nonlinearity is revealed in four main ways: (1) by the nonlinear growth of cochlear responses with stimulus intensity, (2) by the reduction in the response to one stimulus by a second stimulus ('two-tone suppression'), and (3) by the generation of combination tones, or in other words intermodulation distortion products.

5.6.1 The nonlinear growth of cochlear responses

Figure 3.13A shows that basilar membrane responses grow nonlinearly with intensity, for stimulus frequencies around the characteristic frequency. The figure shows that for stimulus frequencies between 9 and 11 kHz and for stimulus amplitudes greater than 30 dB SPL, the amplitude function has a slope of approximately 0.3 on log–log scales, indicating that basilar membrane vibration grows in proportion to the stimulus amplitude raised to the power of 0.3.

The nonlinearity arises from the active mechanical amplification of the travelling wave which starts to saturate or reach its maximum output, by about 30–40 dB SPL. Such saturation of the active component is shown by the solid line in Fig. 5.24. The overall amplitude function of the basilar membrane response can therefore be separated into two parts:

(1) A nearly linear growth up to about 30 dB SPL, which is dependent on an approximately linear growth of the outer hair cell input–output functions and hence of the active mechanical process
(2) A saturating function up to 80–100 dB SPL, which is dependent on the saturation of the hair cell response

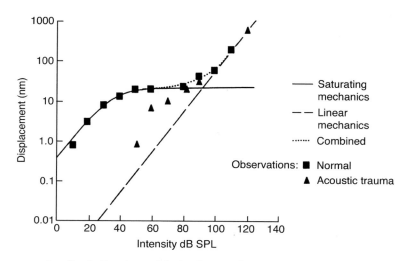

Fig. 5.24 Amplitude functions of the basilar membrane, showing theoretical contributions from the active process (solid line) and the passive process (long dashes), making a net function shown by the dotted line. ■, Measured basilar membrane response when cochlea in good condition. ▲, Measured response after acoustic trauma. Not all investigators have shown the second high-intensity linear phase plotted here. Reprinted from Johnstone *et al.* (1986), Fig. 5, Copyright (1986), with permission from Elsevier.

Some investigators have also shown a further phase of linear growth at the highest stimulus intensities, in cases where the linear passive component has become larger than the active component (see Fig. 5.24). The saturating function is seen only around and above the characteristic frequency, because it is only here that the active process is dominant.

Noise trauma might be expected to impair a physiologically active process, and amplitude functions made before and after the induction of noise trauma show a change from the initial three-part function to one that more closely approximates a simple linear growth (see Fig. 5.24, triangles). Analogous results are seen with the many manipulations that can be expected to affect the active mechanical amplification that linearize the intensity functions as well as making cochlea less sensitive (see, e.g., Fig. 3.13, dashed lines).

Why does the active contribution start to saturate at such a low stimulus intensity? The saturation could occur at two possible stages: (1) saturation of the transducer current as a function of stereociliar displacement and (2) saturation of the motile mechanism as a function of transducer current.

The evidence suggests that saturation of mechanotransduction is likely to be the dominant factor. As described above, manipulation of the stereocilia on all types of hair cells, including outer hair cells, shows that transducer current is limited at larger deflections (see Fig. 3.20). We also expect the responses to rise nearly linearly at very low stimulus intensities, because the hair cell input–output functions have a short approximately linear region around their midpoints.

The motile process from outer hair cells is therefore expected to be initially nearly linear and then saturate. Basilar membrane responses will then show a similar pattern of non-linearity, because outer hair cell transduction saturates (Russell et al., 1986a,b). The form of the saturation can therefore be directly related to the kinetics of mechanotransducer gating, and hence to the Boltzmann function, since this underlies the input–output function of hair cells (see Fig. 5.13).

While the cell body-based motile process is also non-linear, the degree of non-linearity is probably not enough to contribute to the overall non-linearity of the response (Santos-Sacchi, 1993). Stereociliar-based motility is likely to share the non-linear properties of the mechanotransduction with which it is so closely related.

Because the outer hair cells in the basal turn do not show d.c. responses with low intensities of stimulation, it can be concluded that in vivo the outer hair cells are biased towards the central part of the input–output functions, i.e. to the point around which the function is most symmetrical. Because their stereocilia are embedded in the tectorial membrane, the hair cells' zero point is influenced by the zero position of the cochlear partition as a whole. This suggests that the zero point is set to within a few tens of nanometres, extraordinary for a structure that is one hundred or more micrometres wide. This further suggests that the point must be set actively, i.e. the outer hair cells detect a shift from the central position and, by mechanisms that are not certain, act to correct it. This is an issue that has been subject to speculation without resolution for many years. Some possible mechanisms are adaptation, which in outer hair cells can shift the input–output function by at least 50 nm (see Fig. 5.14B), the fast somatic motile mechanism, which can generate movements of up to 1 μm in basal turn outer hair cells, or slow somatic motility (Zenner et al., 1985). It was earlier speculated that a reflex arc via the Type II afferents from the outer hair cells, to the brainstem, and back to the outer hair cells via the medial olivocochlear bundle could affect the static position of the basilar membrane; however, Murugasu and Russell (1996) found that stimulation of the olivocochlear bundle affected only the oscillatory, and not the static, position of the basilar membrane.

5.6.2 Two-tone suppression

It was described in Chapter 4 how the presence of one stimulus can reduce the response of the cochlea to other stimuli. Figure 4.15A shows the tuning curve for the suppressive effect when the suppressed tone ('probe') is set to the nerve fibre's characteristic frequency and the suppressing tone is moved in frequency. The explanation given in Chapter 4 for two-tone suppression was the following: because of the saturating input–output functions of the outer hair cells, each stimulus will push the response to the other into the flatter part of the input–output function. This means that each stimulus will reduce the active amplification of the other's mechanical travelling wave (as well as of course reducing the active amplification of its own travelling wave, revealed in the saturation of basilar membrane mechanics).

Further evidence on the possible mechanism of two-tone suppression has been produced by measuring the mechanical response of the basilar membrane to a high-frequency stimulus at the characteristic frequency of the region, while presenting an intense tone of very low frequency. The excursions of the low-frequency tone displace the outer hair cells to the ends of their operating ranges, suppressing the mechanical response to the characteristic frequency tone twice per cycle (e.g. Geisler and Nuttall, 1997). The major phase of suppression was seen when the basilar membrane was displaced towards the scala tympani, with a second smaller phase of suppression during displacements towards the scala vestibuli.

Similar effects have been seen in the tuning curves of inner hair cells, made during different phases of the intense low-frequency tone. The tuning curves moved upwards and increased in width during the suppressive phases, with the greatest effect being seen during deflections to the scala tympani (Fig. 5.25; Patuzzi

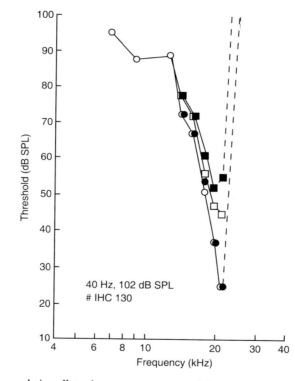

Fig. 5.25 Inner hair cell tuning curves, measured during the different phases of a simultaneous low-frequency stimulus. The tuning curve is sharpest at the moments at which the low-frequency stimulus is going through its zero crossings (○●) and broader and of higher threshold during the extremes of movement towards the scala tympani (■) and the scala vestibuli (□). The tuning curves were made for d.c. receptor potentials of 0.9 mV. Reprinted from Patuzzi and Sellick (1984), Fig. 3, Copyright (1984), with permission from Elsevier.

system, these features do not appear to be as clearly and as separately extracted and encoded in readily definable stages, as are the basic features in the visual system.

A second theme is the localization of functions to the activity of individual cells. In the context of feature detection, it involves finding cells that respond to specific features, so that the detection of a feature can be defined by the activity of single cells studied in isolation. At the other end of a continuum, detection might only be defined by the pattern of activity over many cells. In a common analogy, the first case might be compared to a photograph, in which each point on the photograph represents one point in space, whereas the opposite end of the continuum might be compared to a hologram, in which each point on the hologram represents many points in space, and in which individual points in space can be reconstructed only by the integration of information from many points on the hologram. It is likely many of the more complex features will only be represented in the second form, and at any level of the auditory system, we might expect to find many coexisting stages in between the two extremes.

A third theme is that of hierarchical processing, in which successively more complex analyses are performed at ascending levels of the nervous system, and in which analysis of more complex features is based on an earlier analysis of more simple features.

Schemes for sensory analysis based on the logical extremes of each of the three themes – that is, on the extraction of specific features, on the representation of the features in the activity of single cells, and on hierarchical analysis of features – naturally spring to mind. But it seems that the auditory system operates far from these logical extremes at least on the first two points. For instance, a feature may be represented only in a pattern of activity across many cells, with different patterns of activity within the same population of cells representing different features. Such a mode of operation has contributed greatly to the difficulty of the electrophysiological analysis of the central auditory nervous system.

The likely reason is that many of the critical features of the acoustic stimulus are intermingled in the stimulus, and the neural extraction of some of the features degrades the neural representation of other features. As an example, sound localization that is based on interaural timing requires the preservation of precise time information. However, neuronal circuits that extract the features of complex spectra degrade time information. These two aspects of the stimulus cannot therefore be simultaneously extracted in the same neural circuit: the nervous system extracts them in separate circuits and combines the information at a later stage. This means that extraction of a number of features has to occur in separate parallel systems, with the results being integrated at one or more later stages. When the recombination occurs, the different features are resynthesized to form a neural representation of the auditory properties of the object that gave rise to them, that is, they begin to define what has been called an 'auditory object.'

The result is that, as we move through the auditory system, we see a progressive enhancement of the different features over many stages, with the gradual emphasis of, for instance, spectral contrast, temporal fluctuations and sound location, being built up over multiple stages of the system, and being represented in separate functional channels. At the later stages where the resynthesis occurs (particularly in the inferior colliculus and beyond), the neurones become driven by multiple and selected aspects of the features that were strongly represented in the earlier channels.

Analysis of feature extraction in the central auditory pathway suggests a general division into different functional streams at an early stage. At the cochlear nucleus, two streams are already visible, one of which is involved in binaural sound localization, and the other of which is predominantly involved in sound identification, although with some involvement in sound localization. The information from these streams is then progressively recombined in the higher nuclei, namely in the nuclei of the lateral lemniscus, the inferior colliculus and the medial geniculate body.

A different type of functional division is also visible in the auditory pathway. Both the streams, mentioned above, are parts of the specific, core, or lemniscal auditory system. This can be distinguished from a non-specific, diffuse, extra-lemniscal, or belt system, which is concerned with auditory reflexes and multi-modal integration. The nuclei of this system are the nuclei surrounding the central nucleus of the inferior colliculus, the dorsal and medial divisions of the medial geniculate body, and the secondary and association auditory cortices. This system receives a heavy input from the dorsal cochlear nucleus which, as well as being part of the specific auditory system, could for this reason also be said to be the first stage of the non-specific auditory system.

6.2 THE COCHLEAR NUCLEI

6.2.1 Output pathways

In view of the diversity of the properties of cochlear nucleus neurones, anatomical studies are vital in aiding physiologists in analysing the functions of the nuclei. Classification of the different cells, firstly by linking physiological responses with anatomical cell type, and then by analysing the cells in terms of their output connections, has permitted a straightforward link to be made between anatomy and function.

Cells of the cochlear nucleus project to higher nuclei through two main streams (Fig. 6.11). Cells that project via a ventral stream, running in the trapezoid body on the ventral surface of the brainstem, primarily project to the superior olivary nuclei of the two sides. Here, the timings and intensities of the stimuli at the two ears are compared, and the information is used for sound localization. This pathway forms the binaural sound localization stream. Cells that project via a more dorsal stream, in the dorsal and intermediate acoustic striae, project mainly to the contralateral nuclei of the lateral lemniscus and inferior colliculus. They are mainly involved in the complex analysis of auditory stimuli, forming a stream mainly subserving sound identification.

6.2.2 Input pathways

Each fibre of the auditory nerve branches on entering the nucleus, sending one branch rostrally and the other caudally. The rostral or anterior branch carries fusiform cells, if the rising edge of the notch is at or near the best frequency of the cell (Reiss and Young, 2005). In this case, the stimulus energy just above the upper edge of the notch falls in the excitatory response area of the cell. Such notches in the spectra of broadband stimuli are produced by the transformation of sound field by the pinna (Fig. 2.2B). We would therefore expect the fusiform cells to be responsive to the elevation of broadband sound sources, which are judged on the basis of pinna-derived spectral cues. This agrees with behavioural data, because after lesions of the dorsal acoustic stria, the output pathway of the fusiform cells, cats are less able to make reflex orientations to sound sources as a function of elevation (Sutherland *et al.*, 1998a; May, 2000).

The deficit described by Sutherland *et al.* (1998a) was one to reflexive orientation, in which the cats made an automatic unlearned movement of the head upwards towards a sound source at different elevations. This response was upset by lesions that included the dorsal and intermediate acoustic striae. In contrast, after similar lesions, cats could still learn to *discriminate between* sound sources at different elevations, using a behavioural conditioning task (Sutherland *et al.*, 1998b). In other words, it is the automatic reflexive nature of the response that was critical for the deficit found by Sutherland *et al.* (1998a). This suggests that the dorsal nucleus might be part of an automatic reflex circuit. The ventral pathway, which of course also contains information on the spectrum of the sound, might in contrast be used for behaviour that is learned. It has been in fact speculated that the dorsal cochlear nucleus has much in common with the cerebellum, also involved in automatic motor activity (Oertel and Young, 2004).

6.3 THE SUPERIOR OLIVARY COMPLEX

6.3.1 Innervation and overall anatomy

The outflows from the cochlear nucleus can be divided into two main streams. A binaural sound localization stream runs ventrally in the ventral acoustic stria. A dorsal stream, which is mainly involved in sound identification, runs near the dorsal surface of the brainstem in the dorsal and intermediate striae (Fig. 6.11).

The binaural sound localization stream runs ventrally to the superior olivary nuclei of both sides (Fig. 6.12). The stream has two divisions. In the first division, the intensities of the stimuli at the two ears are compared in the lateral superior olive (LSO). The fibres to the ipsilateral LSO run directly to the nucleus, while those to the contralateral LSO project via synapse in the contralateral medial nucleus of the trapezoid body (MNTB). The second division compares the timings of the stimuli at the two ears. This comparison is undertaken in the medial superior olive (MSO). The fibres from the AVCN project directly to the MSOs of both sides without an intervening synapse.

The dorsal stream, mainly involved in sound identification, runs primarily to the inferior colliculus of the opposite side, some fibres synapsing in the nuclei of

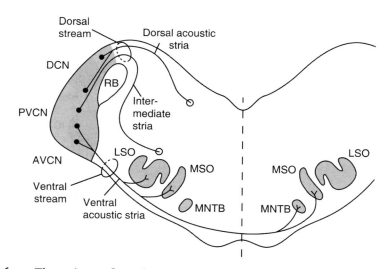

Fig. 6.11 The major outflows from the cochlear nucleus are shown on a transverse section of the cat brainstem. The ventral stream (binaural sound localization stream) arises in the anteroventral cochlear nucleus (AVCN) and posteroventral cochlear nucleus (PVCN) and runs in the ventral acoustic stria to the superior olivary nuclei of both sides (see Fig. 6.8 for further details). The dorsal stream (mainly sound identification stream) runs in the dorsal and intermediate acoustic striae and passes dorsally over the restiform body (RB), or inferior cerebellar peduncle. It arises in the dorsal cochlear nucleus (DCN) and PVCN. Most fibres of the dorsal stream leave the plane of the section (shown by small circles) to run to higher levels of the brainstem, while others (not shown) run to the cells surrounding the lateral superior olive (LSO). MSO, medial superior olivary nucleus; MNTB: medial nucleus of the trapezoid body. Other fires (not shown) run between the cochlear nuclei of both sides. The fibres are represented diagrammatically and do not necessarily branch or join as indicated. For this diagram, anterior sections containing the AVCN and more posterior sections containing the PVCN and DCN have been superimposed.

the lateral lemniscus on the way. Many of the fibres in the intermediate acoustic stria arise from the octopus cells and project to the contralateral VNLL, with some also projecting to the nuclei surrounding the LSO and MSO, or the peri-olivary nuclei.

Within the superior olivary complex itself, several subnuclei can be distinguished (Fig. 6.13), all receiving different distributions of fibres from the different regions of the cochlear nuclei. The main nuclei associated with the ascending auditory pathways are the lateral and medial nuclei of the superior olive (LSO and MSO), and the medial nucleus of the trapezoid body (MNTB). These nuclei are surrounded by other nuclei, known as the pre-olivary and peri-olivary nuclei, which send connections to the other olivary nuclei, as well as being associated with the centrifugal auditory system. They will be discussed in Chapter 8.

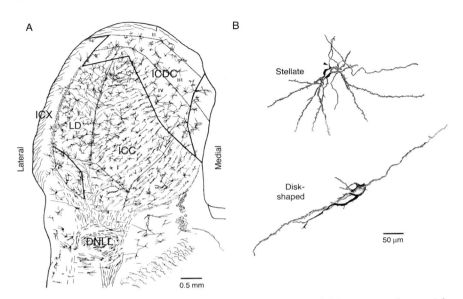

Fig. 6.20 (A) Drawing of the inferior colliculus from Golgi-impregnated material, showing divisions of the nucleus according to Morest and Oliver (1984), and the lamination in part of the central nucleus (ICC). LD, lateral division of central nucleus. I–IV, layers of dorsal cortex. ICDC, dorsal cortex of inferior colliculus; ICX, external nucleus of inferior colliculus; DNLL, dorsal nucleus of the lateral lemniscus; LD, lateral division of ICC. (B) Large disk-shaped cell of the central nucleus, see edge-on as in transverse sections, plus a simple stellate cell, seen in same plane of section as the disk-shaped cell. Arrowhead: axon of stellate cell. A from Morest and Oliver (1984), Fig. 2; B from Oliver and Morest (1984), Figs 1C and 3C, Copyright (1984) Journal of Comparative Neurology reprinted with permission of Wiley-Liss, Inc., a subsidiary of John Wiley & Sons, Inc.

LSO, the ipsilateral MSO, and 30% of the cells of the ipsilateral VNLL. Those inputs are presumed to be glutamatergic as well as using other excitatory amino acids as neurotransmitters. The major ascending inhibitory inputs arise from the DNLL bilaterally (GABAergic), the ipsilateral LSO (glycinergic) and the ipsilateral VNLL (GABAergic and glycinergic). About 30% of the intrinsic neurones of the ICC are GABAergic. They would be able to act as interneurones and provide inhibition within the nucleus via their collateral axons, as well as sending inhibitory projections to the medial geniculate body (Oliver et al., 1994; Winer et al., 1996; Merchan et al., 2005). In addition, there is an input from the contralateral inferior colliculus (not shown in Fig. 6.21).

6.5.2.2 Patterns of excitation and inhibition

In anaesthetized animals, the majority of neurones in the ICC have sharp tuning curves, while a minority have long, shallow, low frequency tails to the curves

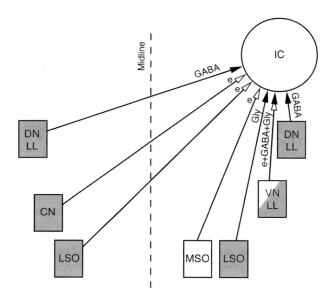

Fig. 6.21 The main ascending excitatory (open arrows) and inhibitory (closed arrows) pathways to the central nucleus of the inferior colliculus. Nuclei sending a predominantly inhibitory input are shown shaded. Some nuclei (e.g. VNLL) send a mixed input. Many minor ascending pathways, and all descending pathways, are not shown. In addition, there is an innervation from the contralateral inferior colliculus (IC). For the inhibitory pathways, the main neurotransmitter is shown. CN, cochlear nucleus; DNLL, dorsal nucleus of the lateral lemniscus; e, excitatory neurotransmitter; gly, glycine; LSO, lateral superior olive; MSO, medial superior olive; VNLL, ventral nucleus of the lateral lemniscus. Data on neurotransmitters and projections from DNLL, Adams and Mugnaini (1984); LSO, Glendenning *et al.* (1992); MSO, Helfert *et al.* (1989); VNLL, Riquelme *et al.* (2001).

(Fig. 6.22A and B). In unanaesthetized animals, the response areas can be more complex in some neurones, with more than one excitatory area and multiple areas of inhibition (Ramachandran *et al.*, 1999; Fig. 6.22C). Where inhibitory areas flank the excitatory area, this forms an example of lateral inhibition. In some neurones, the inhibitory areas stop the excitatory area widening at higher stimulus intensities, so that sharp tuning maintained at all intensities. In some cases, this is so extreme that the excitatory response area disappears at the highest intensities, giving a so-called closed excitatory response area, while in others there may be an inhibitory island within the excitatory response curve (Alkhatib *et al.*, 2006).

The inhibition within the ICC may arise from either the inhibitory inputs to the nucleus or the inhibitory collaterals of the intrinsic neurones of the ICC. In neurones with simple V-shaped response areas (Fig. 6.22A), blocking the inhibition increases neuronal firing to a similar extent both in the central excitatory part of the response area and in the inhibitory flanks. Therefore in these cells, the inhibitory synapses on cells of the ICC tend to affect the whole response area equally and do nucleus (Kwon and Pierson, 1997). Following activation of the inferior colliculus, activity spreads to the reticular formation, the superior colliculus and basal ganglia (for reviews, see Faingold, 1999; Ross and Coleman, 2000). Audiogenic seizures have become a valuable general model for analysing epilepsy and for studying the effects of anti-convulsant medication and neuronal implants.

6.7.2 Learned responses

The modification of auditory-evoked responses as a result of training has been reported in all the stages of the auditory system from the cochlea onwards. It is hazardous to interpret these changes in terms of local neuronal plasticity, because of the problems of stimulus variability in a freely moving animal, and because the auditory input at any one stage can be controlled by multiple efferent or centrifugal mechanisms, under the influence of the animal's central state. These efferent mechanisms start right in the sound conductive pathway, with the middle ear muscles which can affect transmission through the middle ear, and are present at every stage thereafter.

Reliable local changes in neuronal responsiveness during associative conditioning (in which a previously neutral auditory stimulus is paired with a usually aversive unconditioned stimulus, such as a foot shock) are first seen in the medial geniculate body, and in particular in its medial and dorsal divisions (e.g. Birt et al., 1979; O'Connor et al., 1997). Training enhances the synaptic efficacy of the inputs, as it enhances the responses of cells in the medial division to electrical stimulation of the auditory input pathway, which runs in the brachium of the inferior colliculus. The synaptic efficacy of this input could be enhanced, even though response to a control input, from the superior colliculus, was not affected (McEchron et al., 1996).

Synaptic efficacy is commonly modulated via glutamate receptors of the N-methyl-D-aspartate type. Local injection of a selective NMDA antagonist to the recording site in the medial MGB reduces the response to stimulation of the brachium of the inferior colliculus, suggesting that NMDA receptors are involved (Webber et al., 1999). In addition, chemical stimulation of the NMDA receptors enhances the excitability of neurones in the medial MGB and increases the post-synaptic response to the neural input (Ran et al., 2003). These results suggest a neuronal mechanism by which auditory transmission through the medial MGB might be modifiable.

The medial MGB (together with the posterior intralaminar nucleus) sends projections to the amygdala, a nucleus that is involved in the recognition of fearful stimuli and in fear conditioning. The projections go first to the lateral amygdala and then to the basal amygdaloid nuclei and then to the central nucleus. Small lesions of the lateral amygdala, or of the medial MGB plus posterior intralaminar nucleus, interrupt fear conditioning to an auditory stimulus (LeDoux et al., 1990). The lateral amygdala is a major site of plasticity in the conditioning of fear to an auditory stimulus, although it is likely that plasticity in the medial MGB and posterior intralaminar nucleus is involved as well (for reviews, see Maren and Quirk, 2004, and Rodrigues et al., 2004).

6.8 Summary

1. The analysis of auditory stimuli is progressively undertaken over many stages of the auditory system, where the critical features are progressively extracted to a greater and greater extent as the information is passed up the auditory pathway. The likely reason is that many of the critical features of the acoustic stimulus are intermingled in the stimulus, such that the neural extraction of some of the features degrades the neural representation of other features. This means that extraction of a number of features has to occur in separate parallel streams, with the results being integrated at one or more later stages. When the recombination occurs, the responses to the different features are resynthesized to form a neural representation of the auditory properties of the object that gave rise to them, that is, they begin to define what has been called an 'auditory object'.

2. The auditory system shows an early division into two streams with broadly different functions, forming a stream involved in binaural sound localization and a stream predominantly involved in sound identification. At the level of the cochlear nucleus, the binaural sound localization stream involves the anteroventral cochlear nucleus and some cells of the posteroventral cochlear nucleus, which project ventrally over the brainstem in the trapezoid body to the superior olivary complex of both sides. Here, the location of sound sources in the horizontal direction is extracted on the basis of interaural timing and intensity cues. The stream predominantly involved in sound identification includes other cells of the posteroventral cochlear nucleus and dorsal cochlear nucleus and projects directly to the contralateral ventral nucleus of the lateral lemniscus and the contralateral inferior colliculus.

3. The cochlear nucleus has three divisions, known as the anteroventral, posterovental and dorsal cochlear nuclei. Each division of the nucleus is tonotopically organized, so that the best frequencies of the neurones make a spatially ordered map in each division. In the anteroventral division, the neuronal responses are similar to those of auditory nerve fibres, with simple tuning curves, no inhibitory sidebands and monotonic rate–intensity functions. Globular and spherical bushy cells predominate, each receiving synaptic terminals of the auditory nerve fibres in the form of a few large end bulbs of Held, giving fast and secure activation of the neurones. They project to the superior olivary complex via the ventral, binaural sound localization, stream.

4. In the posterovental cochlear nucleus, as well as globular bushy cells, there are octopus cells, which have broad tuning curves and fast temporal responses. Octopus cells can follow the temporal variations in broadband stimuli up to high rates. The cells project via the dorsal predominantly sound identification pathway, primarily to the contralateral ventral nucleus of the lateral lemniscus. The posteroventral cochlear nucleus also contains stellate cells (also present in the anteroventral nucleus). Stellate cells (also known as multipolar cells) are of two types, the more numerous T-stellate cells and the less numerous D-stellate cells. T-stellate cells project bilaterally to the inferior colliculus and

to the ventral nucleus of the lateral lemniscus as well as to the cochlear nucleus and superior olive. D-stellate cells send inhibitory collaterals widely within the cochlear nuclei.

5. The dorsal cochlear nucleus has multiple cell types, the major output cells being the fusiform cells. Cells of the dorsal nucleus tend to have very complex tuning curves, strong bands of inhibition and non-monotonic rate-intensity functions. Cells of the dorsal nucleus, as well as projecting within the nucleus, project via the dorsal stream which is predominantly involved in sound identification to the contralateral inferior colliculus. Some of the cells of the dorsal nucleus respond well to spectral notches and may be involved in judging the elevation of sound sources based on spectral cues introduced by the pinna. Many cells in the cochlear nucleus emphasize spectral contrast and temporal fluctuations in the stimulus.

6. The superior olivary complex receives an input from the anteroventral and posteroventral cochlear nuclei. The superior olivary complex has several component nuclei. The largest component nucleus, the lateral superior olive (LSO), receives an input from both sides, the ipsilateral input being excitatory and the contralateral input inhibitory, via a synapse in the medial nucleus of the trapezoid body. The nucleus is therefore responsive to differences in interaural sound intensity. It is mainly a high-frequency nucleus and uses the differences in interaural sound intensity and time of arrival of transients in the stimulus to code the direction of mainly high-frequency sound sources, being most strongly driven by sound sources on the ipsilateral side of the head. Another component nucleus, the medial superior olive, is mainly a low-frequency nucleus. It is responsive to differences in interaural timing and uses these to code the direction of low frequency sound sources in space, being most strongly driven by sound sources on the contralateral side of the head.

7. The projections from the superior olivary complex, and some of the projections from the cochlear nucleus, travel to the inferior colliculus in the tract known as the lateral lemniscus. Some of the fibres in the tract synapse in the dorsal and ventral nuclei of the lateral lemniscus. The ventral nucleus of the lateral lemniscus (VNLL) is part of the sound identification stream. Its anatomical structure has a complex patchiness which suggests that it contributes complex cross-frequency interactions to the inferior colliculus. The dorsal nucleus of the lateral lemniscus (DNLL) is part of the sound localization stream and enhances the lateralization of stimuli in the auditory system. The fibres within the lateral lemniscus and from the VNLL and DNLL project to the inferior colliculus in such a way that neurones in the colliculus, and in all stages in the auditory system thereafter, predominantly represent sound sources on the contralateral side of the head.

8. The inferior colliculus marks a jump in the complexity of the responses. Here, the results of the analyses that were undertaken in separate streams at the lower levels of the auditory system are combined to give responses that begin to define an auditory object. The inferior colliculus has three main divisions,

namely a central nucleus (the specific, core or lemniscal auditory relay) and two non-specific, diffuse, belt, or extra-lemniscal nuclei, called the dorsal cortex and external nucleus. The central nucleus has a pronounced laminar structure, with the lamina corresponding to isofrequency planes, otherwise known as frequency-band laminae. The nucleus receives a multiplicity of excitatory and inhibitory inputs from the lower auditory nuclei. A great variety of response types are seen in the central nucleus, with some very sharp and some very wide tuning curves. Many cells show enhanced responses to temporal fluctuations, and most neurones are responsive to the location of sound sources. There is evidence that some of these properties are distributed differentially and in patches across each frequency-band lamina. Neurones in the less specific external nucleus and dorsal cortex are often broadly tuned and tend to habituate rapidly. Neurones in the external nucleus commonly respond to the directions of sound sources and often have multimodal responses (e.g. to auditory and somatosensory stimuli). The external nucleus is therefore likely to be an auditory and somatosensory integrative area, governing among other things spatial reflex responses to sound.

9. The medial geniculate body is the specific thalamic relay of the auditory system, receiving afferents from the inferior colliculus and projecting to the auditory cortex. It has three divisions, namely the ventral, dorsal and medial divisions. The ventral division is the specific, core, or lemniscal auditory relay and projects to the primary auditory cortex. It has a laminar structure, where individual adjacent laminae are likely to be organized together into functional units called 'slabs'. The ventral division further sharpens frequency resolution and in species with auditory specializations performs further analyses related to those specializations. It also has heavy reciprocal connections with the auditory cortex and must be seen as a functional unit with the cortex. The medial and dorsal divisions of the medial geniculate body form part of the non-specific, diffuse, belt, or extra-lemniscal auditory system. The later divisions project widely to the areas of cortex surrounding the primary auditory cortex, have multimodal interactions (i.e. visual and somatosensory as well as auditory) and have responses that are modifiable as a result of learning.

10. Unlearned brainstem auditory reflexes include (i) the middle ear muscle reflex, which involves a reflex arc of 2–4 neurones, starting at the cochlear nucleus and going to the motor nuclei of the facial and trigeminal nerves, either directly or via the superior olive; (ii) acoustic startle, which is a reflexive contraction of the muscles of the head and neck and which uses a projection from the ventral cochlear nucleus to a nucleus in the reticular formation, the nucleus reticularis pontis caudalis; (iii) reflexive orientation to auditory stimuli, which involves the external nucleus of the inferior colliculus and the superior colliculus; (iv) audiogenic seizures which depend on the inferior colliculus, especially its external nucleus and dorsal cortex. The seizures arise from a hypersensitivity of the auditory system, probably in these nuclei, that develops in certain susceptible strains of animals in response to early auditory deprivation.

11. The medial geniculate body is the lowest level of the auditory system which is reliably modifiable by learning. The changes particularly occur in the medial and dorsal divisions of the geniculate and occur as a result of activation of NMDA receptors. The medial division also has close links with the lateral amygdala, a pathway which is involved in fear conditioning to an auditory stimulus.

6.9 FURTHER READING

Volumes in the Springer Handbook of Auditory Research (Pub. Springer: series editors R.R. Fay and A.N. Popper) deal with the auditory subcortical areas. The older literature was reviewed in Volumes 1 and 2 ('The Mammalian Auditory Pathway: Neuroanatomy', 1992, and 'The Mammalian Auditory Pathway: Neurophysiology', 1991). More recent reviews are found in several chapters of Volume 15 'Integrative Functions of the Mammalian Auditory Pathway' (2002; eds D. Oertel, R.R. Fay and A.N. Popper) and Volume 23 'Plasticity of the Auditory System' (2004; eds T.N. Parks, E.W. Rubel, R.R. Fay, and A.N. Popper). The cochlear nucleus has also been reviewed by Young and Oertel (2004). The DNLL was reviewed by Kelly (1997). 'The Inferior Colliculus' (2005; eds J.A. Winer and C.E. Schreiner) has many valuable chapters not only on the inferior colliculus, but on its relation with the rest of the auditory brainstem. The older literature on the auditory brainstem was extensively and thoughtfully reviewed by Irvine (1986). For general reviews of the processing of amplitude modulation in the auditory brainstem, see Frisina (2001) and Joris et al. (2004).

CHAPTER SEVEN

THE AUDITORY CORTEX

The auditory cortex consists of core areas, surrounded by belt and parabelt areas. Auditory stimuli are analysed first in the core areas and then in the belt and the parabelt areas. The core areas and some of the surrounding areas are tonotopically organized, with further patterns of organization (e.g. ear dominance, latency and degree of sensitivity to frequency-modulated stimuli) superimposed on the tonotopic organization. Cells in the auditory cortex can show a wide variety of tuning curves, with either broad or narrow tuning, and single or multiple peaks of frequency sensitivity. They can show specific responses to amplitude- and frequency-modulated stimuli and to the location of sound sources. Neurones show a general progressive increase in complexity of responses from the core to the belt. Behavioural studies suggest that the core auditory cortex is necessary for the response to relatively basic features of the auditory stimulus, such as detecting the direction of frequency change, and for sound localization, while the belt and parabelt areas detect more complex features. It is suggested that the auditory cortex is necessary for the representation of 'auditory objects,' that is, the assembly of information about all auditory features of a stimulus, including its location. It has been speculated that in primates the information is then divided into two general streams, with 'what' information being passed anteriorly in the cerebral cortex and with both 'what' and 'where' information being passed posteriorly and dorsally.

7.1 ORGANIZATION

7.1.1 Anatomy and projections

The auditory areas of the cerebral cortex are divided into core areas, with further surrounding areas. The initial detailed analysis of the auditory cortex was performed in the cat. This was undertaken in accordance with the concepts prevailing at the time, which included a single primary receiving area (AI), plus an adjacent secondary area (AII), and further surrounding 'association' areas. However, later analysis in the cat and in particular the extension of the analysis to a wider range of species including primates has led to a reassessment of this approach. The specific receiving area, which receives its input from the specific or 'lemniscal' ventral division of the medial geniculate body, is now known to contain many areas and is now called the core, while there are multiple adjacent areas, called the belt, and further areas surrounding those, called the parabelt. In many mammalian species, there are believed to be three separate areas with the characteristics of core auditory cortex, and up to eight separate auditory areas in the adjacent belt, with further areas in the parabelt. These multiple cortical representations are thought to contribute to parallel processing of the auditory stimulus, with the different areas preferentially processing selected aspects of the auditory input.

7.1.1.1 Core areas

Core areas of the auditory cortex are defined by a number of criteria. Firstly, the areas can be defined by histological criteria. The cytoarchitectonic appearance of the cortex, determined with Nissl staining which marks the cell bodies and proximal dendrites, shows that the core auditory cortex has the same appearance as the primary sensory cortex for other modalities. Cortex with this appearance is known as 'koniocortex' ('dustcortex'), defined as having a large number of small cells with relatively even packing. Layer IV, which receives the afferent axons, is well developed, while there are no large pyramidal cells, normally the large output cells, in the deepest, output layers. Core sensory cortices also are marked by certain common histochemical characteristics such as a dense reaction for the metabolic enzyme cytochrome oxidase, a dense reaction for the enzyme that deactivates the neurotransmitter acetylcholine (acetylcholinesterase), and a dense reaction for the calcium-binding protein parvalbumin (see Kaas and Hackett, 2000).

Secondly, the core areas have substantial direct inputs from the specific auditory division of the medial geniculate body, that is, from the ventral or 'lemniscal' division. In contrast, the belt or adjacent areas have few or no connections with the specific ventral division, but receive their major inputs from the core auditory areas. They also receive inputs from the non-specific medial and dorsal divisions of the medial geniculate (Winer, 1992; Kaas and Hackett, 2000).

Thirdly, each core area shows a tonotopic organization. A single area is defined as having a single progression of neural characteristic frequencies across the cortical area, from high frequencies to low, or vice versa. Therefore, a progression of characteristic frequencies across an area of cortex that goes from low to high and to low again can be taken as a good indication that the area in fact contains two cortical areas, one for each frequency progression.

The core areas are heavily interconnected by reciprocal connections, and this forms a further criterion by which they are grouped together.

In terms of its cytoarchitecture, core auditory cortex shares some properties with other primary sensory cortex, with six layers and a high density of pyramidal and granule cells in layers II, III and IV, but with sparse staining in layer V (Rose, 1949; see also review by Winer, 1992). In layers II–IV, the cortical cells are organized in vertical columns, separated by zones of dendrites and axons and situated around the periphery of small vertical cylinders 50–60 μm in diameter which are oriented orthogonal to the cortical surface. The columnar arrangement is also visible in human beings, where the cell bodies appear in what have been called a 'rain-shower' formation (Seldon, 1981, Moore and Guan, 2001). The main cells receiving the thalamocortical inputs are pyramidal cells in layers IV and III (Smith and Populin, 2001). This is in contrast with visual cortex, where the main receiving cells are spiny stellate cells. Overall, 25% of the neurones in primary cortex are GABAergic and therefore inhibitory: this proportion rises to 94% for neurones within layer I (Prieto *et al.*, 1994). In contrast, glycine does not appear to be used as an inhibitory neurotransmitter in the auditory cortex (Friauf *et al.*, 1997). Axons and dendrites within AI have substantial patchy lateral ramifications that run across as well as along the frequency-band strips (Matsubara and Phillips, 1988). There is also a particularly rich ramification vertically within each column of cells. Callosal afferents, from the contralateral cortex, similarly ramify vertically within 'callosal columns', that is, within columns of cells having a particularly rich callosal innervation (Code and Winer, 1986).

There are reciprocal connections between the cortical areas and the medial geniculate body, such that cortical activation enhances activity in the region that projects to that area of the cortex and suppresses activity in adjacent areas of the cortex (Zhang and Suga, 1997). The corticofugal fibres also form a way that activity can be transmitted from core cortical areas to other areas (for review, see Smith and Spirou, 2002).

Figures 7.1 and 7.2 show the auditory cortical areas in the cat and macaque. In the cat, areas currently classed as core by the above criteria are the traditional primary auditory cortex AI, the anterior auditory field AAF and the posterior auditory field PAF (Reale and Imig, 1980). In the macaque, the areas most commonly classed as core are the auditory area 1 (AI), the rostral area (R) and the rostrotemporal area (RT). As well as projecting heavily to each other, the core areas project to the adjacent belt areas, but without connections to the more distant auditory fields. The belt areas therefore form an obligatory stage in the output from the core.

7.1.1.2 The belt and parabelt

The belt areas are adjacent to the core. Belt areas are defined by the following criteria: (i) major connections with the dorsal or medial divisions of the medial geniculate, (ii) no or only minor connections with the ventral division of the medial geniculate and (iii) having recordable auditory responses. Each belt area receives inputs from multiple core areas, though with a heavier input from the nearest core area. Therefore, we expect each belt area to have its own separate representation of the cochlea. This is borne out functionally in the macaque, where four of the belt areas have their own frequency progressions (Fig. 7.2).

The macaque parabelt consists of two areas, the rostral and caudal parabelt areas, lateral to the belt. While the core and belt are buried in the lateral sulcus, the parabelt is visible on the lateral surface of the superior temporal gyrus (Fig. 7.2B). The parabelt is defined as an area where injections of tracers give heavy labelling of neurones in the belt, but little in the core (Hackett *et al.*, 1998). It is divided into rostral and caudal halves on the basis of heavier connections of each part with the more rostral and caudal divisions of the belt. Figure 7.3 shows the suggested interconnections of the core, belt and parabelt areas in the macaque. The parabelt also connects to several areas of the frontal lobes, including the frontal eye field, which is involved in directing eye movements.

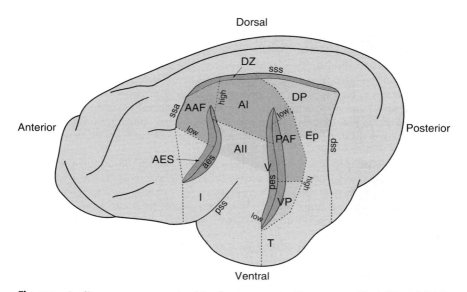

Fig. 7.1 Auditory areas recognized in the cat cortex. Core areas: AI, AAF and PAF. Other areas are belt, surrounded by parabelt. Where the fields are tonotopically organized (AI, AAF, PAF and VP), the representation of highest frequencies (high) and lowest frequencies (low) are marked. Areas shaded darker are hidden in the sulci, which have been opened slightly to show the fields within the sulci. AI, primary auditory cortex; AII, secondary auditory cortex; AAF, anterior auditory field; AES, field of anterior ectosylvian sulcus (buried in sulcus); DP, dorsal posterior area; DZ, dorsal zone, buried on the ventral (lower) surface of the suprasylvian sulcus; Ep, posterior ectosylvian gyrus; I, insula; PAF, posterior auditory field; Sulci, aes and pes, anterior and posterior ectosylvian sulci; pss, pseudosylvian sulcus; ssa and ssp, anterior and posterior suprasylvian sulci; sss, suprasylvian sulcus; T, temporal area; V, ventral field; VP, ventral posterior field. Adapted from Reale and Imig (1980), Fig. 1, including data from Clarey and Irvine (1990), Copyright (1980), Journal of Comparative Neurology reprinted with permission of Wiley-Liss, Inc., a subsidiary of John Wiley & Sons, Inc.

The callosal afferents connect corresponding areas of core, belt and parabelt cortices on the two sides of the brain. There is relatively little cross-over between the different types of cortical area, and this forms an additional criterion by which the areas can be distinguished (Hackett *et al.*, 1999).

7.1.1.3 The human auditory cortex

The position in human beings is less certain, in view of the difficulty of obtaining detailed functional information about sound representation in the human auditory cortex and the substantial variability from one individual to another. Anatomical

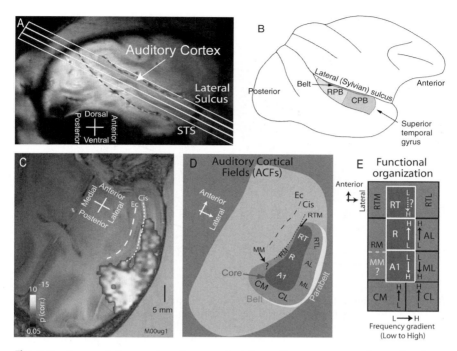

Fig. 7.2 Areas of the monkey (macaque) right auditory cortex as shown by functional magnetic resonance imaging (fMRI). fMRI uses the response to changes in intense magnetic fields to detect activity-related changes in the oxygen depletion of blood. (A) Side view of cortex, showing the planes, through the lower edge of the lateral sulcus, over which images were taken. (B) Diagrammatic representation of the macaque cortex from the same point of view as in part A. The rostral and caudal parabelt areas (RPB, CPB) are shown on the surface of the superior temporal gyrus. (C) Response to broadband noise in one animal. (D) The three core auditory areas (blue) are surrounded by eight belt areas. (E) Tonotopicity of the three core areas and four of the belt areas, shown by representation of high (H) and low (L) frequencies. A1, primary auditory area; AL, anterolateral area; Cis, circular sulcus; CL, caudolateral area; CM, caudomedian area; CPB, caudal parabelt; Ec, external capsule; ML, middle lateral area; MM, middle medial area; R, rostral area; RM, rostromedial area; RPB, rostral parabelt; RT, rostrotemporal area; RTL, lateral rostrotemporal area; RTM, medial rostrotemporal area; STS, superior temporal sulcus. Figure 7.2A, C–E from Petkov *et al.* (2006), Fig. 2. See Plate 1.

studies have therefore been essential for the precise delimitation of the different functional areas.

The auditory cortex is situated on the upper surface of the temporal lobe, on an area known as the superior temporal plane, which is buried within the lateral or Sylvian sulcus or fissure (Fig. 7.4). Because of the depth of the sulcus, and the deep infoldings of the area, the extent of the auditory cortex cannot

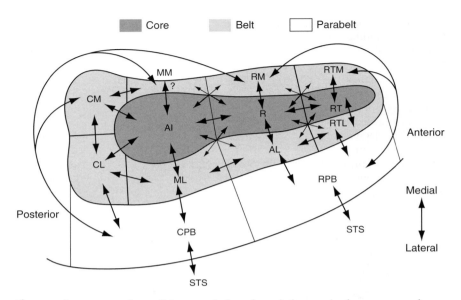

Fig. 7.3 Interconnections of the core, belt and parabelt areas in the macaque, shown on a projection of the upper surface of the superior temporal lobe, according to Hackett *et al.* (1998). Heavy arrows show strong connections, light arrows weaker connections. AL, anterolateral area; CL, caudolateral area; CM, caudomedian area; ML, middle lateral area; MM, middle medial area; R, rostral area; RM, rostromedial area; RPB, rostral parabelt; RTL, lateral rostrotemporal area; RTM, medial rostrotemporal area. From Hackett *et al.* (1998), Fig. 11, Copyright (1998), Journal of Comparative Neurology reprinted with permission of Wiley-Liss, Inc., a subsidiary of John Wiley & Sons, Inc.

be appreciated only from external views. Figure 7.4B shows a surface view of the superior temporal plane once the overlying cortex has been removed and shows a top view of the deep infoldings of the cortical surface on the plane. The primary auditory cortex or core area is situated in the posterior and medial part of Heschl's gyrus, corresponding to Brodmann's area 41 (Brodmann, 1909). The primary cortex is surrounded by several belt and parabelt areas, most of which are also buried within the sulcus. Fig. 7.4C shows a vertical transverse (i.e. coronal) section through the superior temporal plane, and shows the core, belt and parbelt areas of the auditory cortex extending over Heschl's gyrus and laterally over the superior temporal plane to the superior temporal gyrus (see also Fig. 7.4D and E).

The anatomical criteria for the core are the presence of koniocortex and the pattern of cytochrome oxidase and acetylcholinesterase staining. Using Nissl stain, Galaburda and Sanides (1980) identified two distinct divisions within the koniocortex, which they called KAm (medial auditory koniocortex) and KAlt (lateral auditory koniocortex), both of which are likely to be core (Fig. 7.4E). Dense cytochrome oxidase and acetylcholinesterase staining define a similar core area (Rivier and Clarke, 1997; Wallace *et al.*, 2002; Sweet *et al.*, 2005).

Galaburda and Sanides described five further cytoarchitecturally distinct fields in the surrounding cortex which were related to koniocortex, though they were distinguishable from each other in various ways (e.g. by bulkier pyramidal cells in layer III). These are therefore included with the auditory cortex, but are identified as belt and parabelt (Fig. 7.4E; see also Sweet *et al.*, 2005). There is a further area situated more caudally (the temporoparietal area Tpt) which has properties more similar to association cortex than to sensory cortex. Cytochrome oxidase and acetylcholinesterase staining can also be used to define the 5–7 belt areas surrounding the core (Rivier and Clarke, 1997; Wallace *et al.*, 2002; Sweet *et al.*, 2005).

Functional magnetic resonance imaging (fMRI) confirms the presence of auditory responses on the superior surface of the temporal lobe, with a number of separate frequency progression having been found. Talavage *et al.* (2004) found

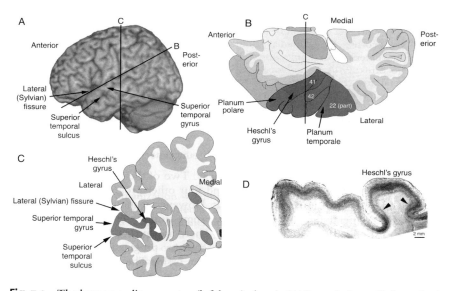

Fig. 7.4 The human auditory cortex (left hemisphere). (A) Lateral view of left cerebral hemisphere, showing planes of section in parts B and C. (B) Sloping section in the plane shown in part A. Top view of upper surface of temporal lobe (red) with area of koniocortex within Heschl's gyrus marked (darker red). The division of the surface anterior to Heschl's gyrus is known as the planum polare, and the large division posterior to Heschl's gyrus is known as the planum temporale. Numbers show areas according to Brodmann (1909). In some individuals, Heschl's gyrus divides into two. (C) Transverse section of left cerebral hemisphere in the vertical plane shown in part A, showing Heschl's gyrus (darker red) and further auditory cortex of the superior temporal plane (lighter red, lighter and darker blue). Exactly how the latter areas are distributed over the superior temporal gyrus and sulcus varies between individuals. (D) Transverse histological section as in part C, showing Heschl's gyrus and laterally adjacent parts of the superior temporal plane. Arrowheads: borders of AI. Nissl stain.

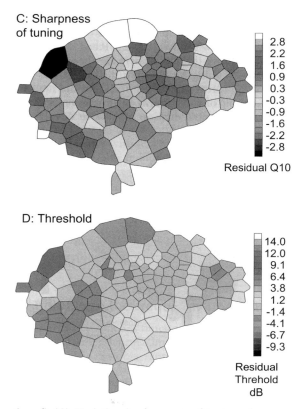

Fig. 7.6 (Continued) (C) Variation in sharpness of tuning: sharpness of tuning was determined near threshold. The 'residual Q10' is the variation from the mean Q10 for that frequency, measured over all cells at that frequency [Q10: a measure of sharpness of tuning, defined as (CF)/(bandwidth of tuning curve measured 10 dB above lowest threshold) see also Chapter 4]. (D) Gradient in thresholds: residual thresholds (threshold of area minus mean threshold of all cells at that CF), shows variation of thresholds in dB. In addition to the groupings shown here, we expect further groupings based on binaural dominance. In Fig. 7.6B–D, the values have been interpolated and smoothed to show trends in spite of the variability from area to area. Used with permission from Cheung *et al.* (2001), Figs 1B, 5B, 11C and 8C. See Plate 4.

responses, while cells in the dorsal division have complex and multi-band response areas. The results suggest that in the cat the central region of AI is involved in analysing narrowband sounds, while the dorsal division is responsible for analysing complex patterns across frequency (Sutter *et al.*, 1999).

The latency of response also varies across the cortex, gradually increasing along each frequency-band strip (shown in the squirrel monkey; Fig. 7.6B; Cheung *et al.*,

2001). Sensitivity to FM also shows organization along the frequency-band strips, cells having high sensitivity to FM tending to be segregated in groups, although with no clear spatial pattern (Heil *et al.*, 1992). It is possible to speculate how the different areas of cells within AI could be specialized for the detection of different aspects of the stimulus, although at the moment the exact details of the different groupings, their interrelation and their functional importance are not clear (for review, see Read *et al.*, 2002).

7.2 THE RESPONSES OF SINGLE NEURONES

7.2.1 Responses in the core

Analysis of the auditory cortex is more difficult than that of lower auditory centres because anaesthesia, and particularly barbiturate anaesthesia, suppresses cortical responses. It reduces spontaneous activity and converts the sustained excitatory and inhibitory responses commonly seen in unanaesthetized animals to transient on or off responses with only a few action potentials per stimulus presentation. However, even in barbiturate-anaesthetized animals, the proportion of responsive neurones has been reported to be as high as 80–90% (e.g. Phillips and Irvine, 1981). In unanaesthetized animals, cells with many different patterns of response are seen in AI, including many cells with sustained and transient responses, and also cells with only on, off or on-off responses, with the most preferred stimuli tending to give the more sustained responses (Abeles and Goldstein, 1972; Wang, 2007).

Most responsive neurones in AI have sharp tuning with a single frequency region of maximum sensitivity (e.g. Phillips and Irvine, 1981). However, some neurones have two or more regions of maximum sensitivity, giving what are known as multipeaked responses (Fig. 7.7A and B). Multipeaked neurones consisted of 20% of the sample recorded by Kadia and Wang (2003) in the unanaesthetized marmoset; in many cases, the peaks were harmonically related to the cell's characteristic frequency (e.g. at twice characteristic frequency, or three times characteristic frequency). Multipeaked neurones are spatially segregated from single peaked neurones, in the cat being found primarily in the dorsal rather than the central region of AI (Sutter and Schreiner, 1991; Schreiner *et al.*, 2000). Other neurones have very broad tuning curves, covering several octaves. In the cat, as in primates, broadly tuned neurones are spatially segregated from those showing sharp tuning.

As in other parts of the auditory system, neurones in AI can be inhibited by stimuli presented outside the excitatory response area, although this can be difficult to detect with single stimuli in cases where neurones have little or no spontaneous activity. In many cases, the inhibitory areas immediately surround the central excitatory area. However in addition, a high proportion of cells can be inhibited by stimuli presented in one or more discrete frequency bands which are remote from the central excitatory or inhibitory area (Sutter *et al.*, 1999; Kadia and Wang, 2003). Some of the inhibition is generated within the cortex, as it can be reduced by the local application of the GABA blocker bicuculline (Wang *et al.*, 2000).

▶ 7.5 OVERVIEW OF FUNCTION OF THE AUDITORY CORTEX

In contrast with earlier results, recent studies have shown deficits in relatively simple functions such as stimulus detection, frequency discrimination and sound localization, after lesions of the auditory cortex. Theories of function for the auditory cortex have therefore moved from previous suggestions that it is only involved in higher level cognitive functions to suggestions that it is also involved in processing stimuli in a more direct way, with stimulus features being first analysed in the core, then in the belt, and then the parabelt.

Responses to complex stimuli suggest that in AI, neurones can respond specifically to sound location, and to stimuli such as multitone complexes, where the cross-frequency interaction is made possible by the neuronal processes that connect across frequency-band strips. The functional pattern of connectivity at any one time would be a combination of genetic programming, the history of exposure of the animal to such stimuli, and the continual moment-by-moment modulations produced by the current demands of the behavioural state of the animal. In this way, the neurones would come to respond to the complex stimuli that are present in the environment, with particular emphasis on those that are of current significance to the animal. Once the stimulus complexes have been analysed in the core areas, the neuronal activity is transferred to the belt, and then the parabelt, where higher and higher levels of analysis are carried out.

It can be hypothesized that the auditory cortex can develop these analyses because not only does its number and range of intrinsic interconnections allow a greater degree of complex interaction than in lower centres, but also because its larger number of neurones, greater degree of plasticity and its non-auditory inputs allow it to adjust its responses to the current demands of the auditory environment and the animal, to a greater extent and in a more complex and subtle way.

The pathways for sound identification and sound location are partially segregated in the early stages of the auditory system, as a result of the different analyses required by the very different acoustic cues for these two aspects of the stimulus (see Chapter 6). Information on identification and location is then progressively combined in the inferior colliculus, medial geniculate body and primary auditory cortex. After this stage, the two types of information are segregated again, into more anterior and more dorsal/posterior pathways, suggested to correspond to hypothetical 'what' and 'where' pathways. This points to the cortex, which is the final stage of convergence of the identification and location streams, and also the first stage of divergence of the 'what' and 'where' streams, as having a special function. It can be hypothesized that in the primary auditory cortex, neuronal activity can be driven specifically by certain auditory objects. Such activity would combine information about the spatial source of the sound derived from the localization pathway, with information about its spectral and temporal nature being derived from the sound identification pathway. Coincidences in the activation of inputs to these neurones during previous auditory experience would facilitate the activation of neurones driven by common combinations of stimuli. This would promote neuronal circuits that could be said to represent the objects. Objects seem to be represented in a pattern of activity over many neurones. Conversely, each neurone may contribute to the representation of many different auditory objects.

The combined information about location and identity is then passed along the hypothetical dorsal/ventral 'where' or 'do' pathway, which responds to both aspects of the stimulus, and which may be involved in preparing the auditory stimulus so that it can be linked with a motor response. In contrast, the 'what' pathway seems to be concerned only with the identity of the stimulus and does not respond to information about location.

7.6 SUMMARY

1. Auditory cortex consists of a core surrounded by a belt and a parabelt. The core contains multiple (e.g. three) areas, including AI. The core receives its major input from the specific or lemniscal division of the thalamic nucleus, namely the ventral division of the medial geniculate body that projects to the auditory cortex. The belt and parabelt areas predominantly receive their inputs from other divisions of the medial geniculate body. The belt also receives intra-cortical projections from the core, and the parabelt receives intra-cortical projections from the belt.

2. Auditory cortical areas are defined by the following criteria: (i) cell types and histological appearance; (ii) connections with the thalamus; (iii) pattern of staining for cytochrome oxidase, acetylcholinesterase and parvalbumin and (iv) the existence of separate tonotopic progressions in some areas.

3. In human beings, the primary auditory cortex is situated in the posterior and medial part of Heschl's gyrus on the superior temporal plane on the upper surface of the temporal lobe, deep in the lateral (Sylvian) sulcus. Belt and parabelt areas surround it rostrally (the planum polare), caudally (the planum temporale) and laterally (the superior temporal gyrus).

4. Primary cortical areas, and some of the belt areas, are tonotopically organized, that is, the characteristic frequencies of neurones change in a progressive manner across the cortex. Lines joining neurones of similar characteristic frequency run orthogonal to the frequency progression and make what are called frequency-band strips. Cells whose responses are dominated by one ear or the other are grouped in patches on the surface of the cortex. Other groupings of cells, not related to the above patterns, can be found when cells are analysed in terms of latency, sharpness of tuning, threshold or sensitivity to frequency modulation. The significance of these groupings is not known.

5. Single neurones in the core areas show many different shapes of tuning curves in response to pure tones. Some neurones have sharp tuning curves with a single frequency region of maximum sensitivity. Others have very broad tuning curves, or 'multipeaked' tuning curves with two or more frequency regions of

maximum sensitivity. Stimuli in the different regions of maximum sensitivity can be facilitatory, so that the neurones are particularly responsive to certain complex stimuli. In many of these cases, the frequencies of maximum sensitivity are harmonically related, so that the neurones would be particularly sensitive to stimuli with a rich harmonic structure, such as vocalizations. In other cases, although only a single excitatory peak is visible in the tuning curve in response to single tones, multiple bands of excitation or inhibition are revealed when further tones are superimposed.

6. Outside AI, in other parts of the core and in the belt areas, neurones seem particularly responsive to complex stimuli, including frequency- and amplitude-modulated tones, with different cortical areas being responsive to different modulation rates.

7. Sound location is represented in the auditory cortex, and unilateral lesions in the auditory cortex interfere with behavioural sound localization on the contralateral side. In the cat, local reversible cooling shows that AI, another core area (PAF) and a belt area (AES) are all essential for behavioural sound localization. In these areas, as well as in other cortical areas, a high proportion of neurones are sensitive to the location of sound sources and use interaural intensity and/or timing as cues.

8. Microelectrode studies in non-human primates, and fMRI in human and non-human primates, suggest that after the core areas, spatial information is processed more caudally and dorsally in the cortex, in what has been called the 'where' or 'do' stream. This includes the posterior temporal gyrus, the inferior parietal cortex and a more anteriorly situated area, near the superior frontal sulcus. On the other hand, complex stimuli particularly activate areas anterior to the auditory core, including in human the planum polare and area around the inferior frontal gyrus. These areas are part of the more rostral 'what' stream. However, there is some crossover and some 'what' information is also represented in the other stream.

9. It is suggested that the role of the auditory cortex in perception is that of representing auditory objects. Different objects are likely to be represented in overlapping patterns of activity spread over many neurones. The pattern of responsiveness of the cortex at any one time reflects the current behavioural state of the animal, with the neuronal responses modifiable such that a larger proportion of cortex is devoted to stimuli of particular current significance.

7.7 FURTHER READING

The anatomy of the auditory cortex has been reviewed by Winer (1992), with more recent updates by Kaas and Hackett (2000), Smith and Spirou (2002) and Winer et al. (2005). Older work on the electrophysiology of the auditory cortex was reviewed by Clarey et al. (1992), while more a recent commentary on cortical function has been given by Semple and Scott (2003). Cortical processing of location and complex stimuli, particularly in relation to single-neurone analysis in animals, has been reviewed by Middlebrooks *et al.* (2002) and by Nelken (2002) respectively, in two chapters of 'Integrative Functions in the Mammalian Auditory Pathway' (Springer Handbook of Auditory Research, Vol. 15, edited by D. Oertel, R.R. Fay, and A. N. Popper), and also by Wang (2007). Complex stimulus processing, particularly in relation to fMRI in human beings, has been reviewed by Griffiths and Warren (2002), Nelken (2004), Scheich *et al.* (2007) and Zatorre (2007). The cortical processing of music has been reviewed by Stewart *et al.* (2006) and Limb (2006). 'What' and 'where' streams have been reviewed by Rauschecker and Tian (2000), with special reference to non-human primates, and by Barrett and Hall (2006) with reference to human beings, with an alternatative view being given by Warren *et al.* (2005). Cortical plasticity has been reviewed by Weinberger (1998, 2004), Ohl and Scheich (2005) and Majewska and Sur (2006).

amplification of the travelling wave, that is, they were not mediated via the MOC. These results suggest that normally the LOC is able to reduce sound-induced damage to the afferent auditory nerve fibres, perhaps by its ability to modify neural responsiveness (see above; see also Chapter 10).

8.2.3.3.2 Improving the detection of signals in noise. Winslow and Sachs (1987) showed that stimulation of the olivocochlear bundle could reduce masking in single auditory nerve fibres. Figure 8.6 shows the rate-intensity functions (solid lines) of an auditory nerve fibre for tone pulses in silence (Fig. 8.6A), and for tone pulses heavily masked by a constant broadband background noise (Fig. 8.6B). In this figure, the firing rates are plotted as a function of tone level. With no olivo-cochlear stimulation, the background noise flattened the tone-intensity function (full line in Fig. 8.6B: compare with full line in Fig. 8.6A). The flattening occurred because, at low tone intensities, the noise itself drove the fibre, and at higher tone intensities, the noise suppressed the response to the tone.

Electrical stimulation of the OCB (dotted line, Fig. 8.6A) shifts the rate-intensity functions for the tone to the right, similar to the effect shown in Fig. 8.4B. However, in the presence of background masking noise, OCB stimulation sup-presses the response to both the noise and the tone. The suppression of the response to the tone shifts its rate-intensity function to the right (dotted line, Fig. 8.6B).

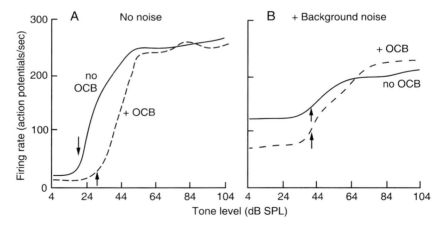

Fig. 8.6 Rate-intensity functions for an auditory nerve fibre, without (————) and with (- - - - -) electrical stimulation of the crossed olivocochlear bundle (OCB). (A) No masking noise. The fibre here is activated only by the tone pulses and shows the standard sigmoidal relation between tone intensity and firing rate. Olivocochlear stimulation shifted the function along the intensity axis by 12 dB. (B) With continuous making noise, the function is flatter (see text). Olivocochlear stimulation reverses the effects and steepens the function. Arrows: point at which the tone increases the firing rate by 20 spikes/sec. For clarity the original published functions have been slightly smoothed. Used with permission from Winslow and Sachs (1987), Fig. 4A and D.

The suppression of the response to the noise by the OCB reduces the extent to which the noise adapts the response to the tone, so that for higher level tones, the response to the tone itself is actually increased. For low-intensity tones, when the noise itself was driving the fibre, the firing of the fibre is reduced. The result is that the rate-intensity function to the tone is steepened as well as being shifted. For stimuli well above threshold, therefore, the OCB stimulation enhanced the response of the fibre to the tone, when in the presence of background noise.

However, the masked detection threshold for the tone in noise was unchanged. As shown in Fig. 8.6, the tone intensity for a small (20 spikes/sec) increment in firing is the same with and without OCB stimulation (arrows, Fig. 8.6B). Kawase *et al.* (1993) confirmed this in more detail in a later experiment and showed that it particularly applied to fibres measured in the presence of relatively low levels of background noise. On the other hand, they found that in some fibres, particularly those with high spontaneous firing rates, and for higher levels of background masking noise, OCB stimulation could lower the detection thresholds of tones in noise, commonly by about 5 dB.

A role in the discrimination of signals in noise was also suggested by the experiments of Dewson (1968). He trained rhesus monkeys to discriminate between two vowel sounds in the presence of masking noise. Performance was reduced by cutting the fibres of the crossed component of the olivocochlear bundle. Similar results have been obtained by Hienz *et al.* (1998) in cats. In human beings, contralateral acoustic stimulation can activate the MOC, as detected by suppression of otoacoustic emissions produced by the ear being tested (for review, see Guinan, 2006). Contralateral stimulation is also able to enhance the detection of tones in noise, likely to occur via an effect on the MOC. For instance, in the experiment of Micheyl and Collet (1996), when the results were averaged over all subjects, contralateral noise did not affect the detection of masked tone pips in the tested ear. However, in those subjects where contralateral noise was particularly effective at suppressing otoacoustic emissions in the tested ear (i.e. presumably those subjects where the crossed MOC reflex was particularly effective), masked thresholds for tone pips in the tested ear tended to be better than in the other subjects, by a few dB. Similar results have been found for the discrimination of speech sounds in noise, with the improvements also being absent in patients in whom the vestibular nerve had been cut, severing all OCB efferents (Giraud *et al.*, 1997).

8.2.3.3.3 *Adjusting the dynamic range of hearing.*

The effects on the intensity functions (Fig. 8.4) and on masking (Fig. 8.6) are both examples of the ways that the OCB can reduce the sensitivity of the auditory system in the presence of intense stimuli. Moderate and intense stimuli can drive auditory nerve fibres into the saturated range of their firing; by reducing the degree of activation of the auditory nerve, the OCB may be able to enhance the dynamic range of the cochlea.

8.2.3.3.4 *Role in attention.*

Could the olivocochlear bundle be involved in attention, attenuating the peripheral response to an auditory signal when it is judged to be irrelevant? Such a hypothesis could explain the common experience the nucleus. The time course of masking was changed in the cochlear nucleus, depending on neurone type, In some types of neurone, the masking of one stimulus by a later stimulus was decreased, while in other types of neurones, the delayed masking was increased, suggesting the removal of either delayed excitation or delayed inhibition on the neurones. It is therefore possible that the centrifugal pathways modify the temporal integration of stimuli in the cochlear nucleus, according to the demands of the task.

8.4 CENTRIFUGAL PATHWAYS IN HIGHER CENTRES

Centrifugal pathways are found at all levels of the auditory system, from cortex to cochlea, with the result that the highest levels of the auditory system are able to influence the lowest (for reviews, see Spangler and Warr, 1991; Smith and Spirou, 2002).

8.4.1 Anatomy
8.4.1.1 Corticofugal system

Two descending systems have been described as originating in the auditory cortex. First, the cortical areas send massive descending projections to the medial geniculate body, particularly to the division from which they receive an ascending innervation. Secondly, the cortex also sends descending projections to a wide range of other areas, including auditory nuclei (the inferior colliculus, the superior olivary complex and the cochlear nucleus) as well as other non–auditory areas, including other nuclei of the thalamus, the tegmentum, the amygdala and the central grey matter, and areas connected to the motor system (for review, see Winer, 2006).

The tonotopic areas of the auditory cortex project primarily to the tonotopic divisions of the medial geniculate, while the non-tonotopic areas project primarily to the non-tonotopic areas of the medial geniculate and to the polymodal areas of the thalamus. Within the tonotopic projections, the descending fibres terminate in a spatially organized way on the cells that project back to the cortex. It seems, therefore, that there is a close coupling in the loop of afferent and efferent fibres, so that each part of the cortex can influence the part of the medial geniculate body that sends it connections, and suggesting that, within each functional division, the thalamus and cortex can act as one unit. In addition to this area-specific projection, there is also a more divergent projection, with each cortical area projecting to multiple areas of the thalamus (Winer *et al.*, 2001).

The cortical projection to the inferior colliculus ends mainly in the external nucleus and dorsal cortex, that is, the extralemniscal areas of the colliculus, which are part of the less specific and sometimes multisensory auditory pathway (Chapter 6). There is also a much smaller projection from the cortex to the superior olivary complex, running mainly ipsilaterally to the ventral nucleus of the trapezoid body (medial preolivary nucleus) and ending on the cells of origin of the MOC (Mulders and Robertson, 2000). The projection to the cochlear nucleus also ends primarily ipsilaterally, in the granule cell layers of all divisions and in all parts of the dorsal nucleus, in particular in its pyramidal (fusiform) layer, ending on cells that project centripetally to the inferior colliculus (Schofield and Coomes, 2005). In addition, the auditory cortex projects to the motor nuclei of the pons, a major source of mossy fibres to the cerebellum, and to the striatum, both of which form parts of the extrapyramidal motor system (Winer, 2006).

8.4.1.2 Centrifugal fibres from inferior colliculus

The inferior colliculus is a further rich source of centrifugal fibres, sending projections to the lateral lemniscus, the superior olivary complex and the cochlear nucleus. The projections to the superior olivary complex end in the ventral nucleus of the trapezoid body and the periolivary region rostral to the nucleus; the centrifugal neurones end on neurones that themselves project to the cochlear nucleus and to the cochlea, the latter via the MOC (Vetter *et al.*, 1993; Schofield and Cant, 1999). The connections from cortex to inferior colliculus and to superior olive, and the olivocochlear bundle to the cochlea, form a way that the cortex can modulate the responses of the cochlea.

8.4.2 Physiology and function

Ma and Suga (2001) recorded from cells in the inferior colliculus of bats, while stimulating in the auditory cortex, within the cortical projection areas of the neurones being recorded from. When the characteristic frequencies of the areas being stimulated and recorded from matched, the neural frequency response areas of the neurones in the lower nuclei became sharpened – that is, the responses to tones at the best frequency were enhanced, and the responses to adjacent frequencies were inhibited. On the other hand, if the characteristic frequencies were unmatched, the stimulation inhibited the response at the characteristic frequency, but enhanced the responses at other frequencies. This shifted the best frequencies of the cells in the lower nuclei, in most cases towards that of the stimulated neurones. The effect is that the cortical activation enhances the responses and sharpens the frequency selectivity of the cells that project to the same area. The direction of the frequency shift in unmatched neurones means that a greater portion of the auditory pathway becomes devoted to the frequencies that are being activated by the cortical stimulation (reviewed by Suga and Ma, 2003). Similar results have been obtained in the mouse by Yan and Ehret (2002). This suggests that centrifugal pathways might be a mechanism by which the cortex can enhance its responses and devote a larger numbers of neurones to stimuli which are of particular current significance for the animal.

The influence of descending fibres from the inferior colliculus can be detected in the responses of the cochlea and auditory nerve, since the fibres end on the cells of origin of the olivocochlear bundle. Mulders and Robertson (2005b) stimulated the inferior colliculus and produced a variety of effects in auditory nerve fibres.

shape (see Unoki *et al.*, 2006). Thus, it has a form generally similar to the frequency filtering functions of auditory nerve fibres, as reflected in their tuning curves. The filter is slightly asymmetric, being wider on the low-frequency side for high-intensity maskers. The asymmetry at high masker levels contributes to the asymmetry of the masking patterns shown in Figs 9.1 and 9.2.

9.3.1.4 Non-simultaneous masking techniques

A technique for measuring frequency resolution that produced a great deal of interest depends on non-simultaneous rather than direct or simultaneous masking (Houtgast, 1977). One technique used by Houtgast was forward masking. In forward masking, the masker is pulsed, each pulse being followed by a brief probe, lasting only 10 or 20 ms. The stimuli are ramped on and off to reduce the effects of spectral splatter. The masker will, of course, raise the threshold of the probe. If the critical band measurements are repeated with forward masking rather than with simultaneous masking a surprising difference emerges: the calculated psychophysical filters necessary to explain the results are commonly rather narrower, and surrounded, particularly on the high-frequency side, by areas of negative transmission. The negative areas can be explained by supposing that they are areas of lateral inhibition or suppression (Fig. 9.3; Houtgast, 1977).

Lateral inhibition or suppression is of course widespread in the auditory system, but had not hitherto been demonstrated convincingly by simultaneous masking

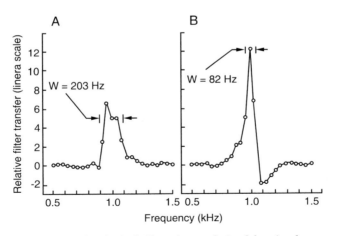

Fig. 9.3 Calculated psychophysical filter shapes derived by simultaneous masking techniques (A) are broader than those determined by non-simultaneous techniques (B). That determined by non-simultaneous masking also has an inhibitory sideband. 'W' indicates the effective bandwidth of the filter, that is, the bandwidth of the equivalent rectangular filter. The filter shapes were calculated from masking the signal with wideband noise which had a rippled spectrum. The frequency spacing and positions of the ripples were varied. Test frequency 1 kHz. Reprinted from Houtgast (1977), Fig. 6, top, Copyright (1977), with permission from American Institute of Physics.

techniques. Houtgast pointed out an obvious reason. We calculate the internal representation of a masker by measuring the threshold of a probe superimposed on the masker. If the elements of a complex masker interact to suppress the masker in some frequency regions, a probe in those frequency regions if presented simultaneously will be suppressed as well and to a similar extent. Because the signal-to-noise ratio is in effect unchanged, the probe threshold will be unchanged, and the suppression areas will not be reflected in the probe threshold. Forward masking acts rather differently. A complex masker will produce regions of high activity and, as a result of lateral suppression or inhibition, some regions of low activity. When the masker is turned off, its after-effects will raise the thresholds of neurones of some later stage in the auditory system, to an extent which depends on the amount of previous activity. If a probe is now presented, its threshold will be raised less in the areas of low activity than in the areas of high activity. In other words, the masking pattern will now reflect the influence of the inhibitory bands as well as that of the excitatory ones. The difference between simultaneous and non-simultaneous masking may reveal the effects only of cochlear nonlinearity, or may include those of neuronal inhibition at later stages as well.

Non-simultaneous masking techniques have generated interest because they can reveal the effects of lateral inhibition. This has suggested that non-simultaneous masking might provide a more accurate picture of the neural representation of auditory stimuli than does simultaneous masking. On the other hand, the detection cues used by the subject in non-simultaneous masking can be more complex than in simultaneous masking, and these can have their own effect on the apparent shape of the filter (Moore and Glasberg, 1982).

9.3.2 Quantitative relations between psychophysics and physiology in frequency resolution

Although it is clear that in general terms psychophysical filters reflect the underlying frequency filtering properties of the auditory system, it is not necessarily the case that the relation holds up quantitatively and in detail. In particular, how closely do psychophysical filters correspond to the frequency resolution of the cochlea, as initially suggested by Fletcher (1940), and as reflected in the frequency filtering properties of auditory nerve fibres?

The tasks used to measure the filters psychophysically depend on interactions between two or more stimuli and are therefore more complex than those used to measure the pure-tone tuning curves of single auditory nerve fibres. In order to establish the correspondence between electrophysiological and psychophysical measures of tuning, the equivalent task must be used in the two cases. One such method is to measure the equivalent of 'psychophysical tuning curves' on individual fibres of the auditory nerve, using a forward masking paradigm analogous to that used psychophysically. In such experiments, a pure-tone tuning curve is first determined for an auditory nerve fibre. The fibre is then excited by tone pips presented at a fixed intensity (e.g. 10 dB above threshold) at the characteristic frequency. As in the conventional psychophysical tuning curve, the response is masked by a tone that is varied in frequency, and adjusted in intensity, so that the constant tone pips techniques which relate the time pattern of firings to the temporal structure of the stimulus waveform can be used to show that the drive to the fibre is still tuned according to the pattern of vibration on the basilar membrane, even though the stimulus intensity is well into the range in which the fibre's firing is saturated (Section 4.2.3).

Is temporal information in fact used in this way to reveal frequency resolution? The auditory nerve does not phase-lock above 5 kHz, so that if performance deteriorates with intensity more above, than below, this frequency limit, the implication is that timing information might be used below the limit. Moore (1975) found that masked thresholds increased with intensity more above than below the 5-kHz frequency limit. Many conceptual models of auditory processing include timing information and obtain matches to psychophysical data that are closer than those obtained using only mean rates of firing (e.g. Colburn et al., 2003; Tan and Carney, 2006). However, it is very difficult to obtain definitive evidence that timing information is actually used in this way.

One type of model uses the temporal relations between the firings in different neural channels to extract information about the stimulus. A simple and physiologically realistic way of doing this, and which enhances rate-place information in the cochlear nucleus, was proposed by Shamma (1985a,b). Shamma pointed out that the relative timing of nerve action potentials in the different fibres of the auditory nerve would be affected by the place of activation along the cochlea. The cochlear travelling wave shows large phase shifts near its peak of vibration. Nerve fibres innervating adjacent regions near the peak will therefore tend to be activated in different phases of the input stimulus. Cells in the cochlear nucleus show lateral inhibition, so that they are excited by nerve fibres innervating one region of the cochlear duct and inhibited by nerve fibres from adjacent regions. If the spatial separation of the excitatory and inhibitory inputs from different parts of the cochlea is suitable, it is possible that excitation will be transmitted in one phase of the stimulus, while the inhibition from adjacent regions is transmitted in the opposite phase. The net effect is that the (opposite) excitatory and inhibitory phases of the waveform will summate, giving large fluctuations of excitation and inhibition in the cell during a cycle of the stimulus (Fig. 9.9). Phase-locked responses in the cell will be thereby enhanced. If the mean firing rate responds non-linearly to changes in membrane potential, the fluctuations will be reflected in an increase in the mean rate.

However, where nerve fibres are activated towards the tail of the travelling wave, where phase changes are smaller as a function of distance, excitation and inhibition will tend to arrive with similar phases at cells of the cochlear nucleus, and the net response of the cell will be small.

Simulations of the model shows that it can preserve the spectral information present in a complex stimulus in the cochlea, over a wide range of intensities, even when the intensity is so high that it has been lost in the mean-rate information in the auditory nerve (Shamma, 1985b).

Other types of model extract timing on the basis of the repetition rates or timing intervals of action potentials within the same, rather than across, neural channels. As pointed out in Section 9.4.2, neural substrates for temporal detection

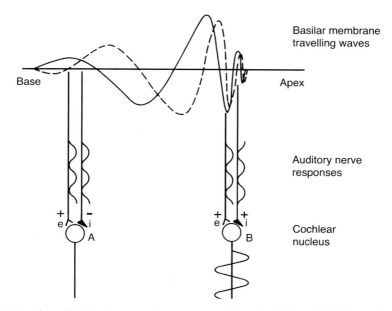

Fig. 9.9 Phase shifts in the travelling wave, combined with lateral inhibitory interactions in the cochlear nucleus, could decode timing information into place information, according to the theory presented by Shamma. Excitatory (e) and inhibitory (i) synapses on neurone A are activated with similar phases, so their effects cancel (+,−). However, excitatory (e) and inhibitory (i) synapses on neurone B are activated in opposite phases, so the responses summate (+,+). Open symbols, excitatory synapses; filled symbols, inhibitory synapses. Reprinted from Shamma (1985a), Fig. 4c, Copyright (1979), with permission from American Institute of Physics.

in the cochlear nucleus, and in particular those depending on the intrinsic temporal properties of chopper cells, are poor. However, as also discussed in Section 9.4.2, some cells of the inferior colliculus may be suitable.

Models incorporating temporal information have two general problems: (i) that of proposing a neural basis for the extraction of the temporal information that is realistic in physiological terms and (ii) obtaining clear and independent physiological evidence that the models are actually valid.

9.5.1.4 The middle ear muscle reflex

Sound-elicited contractions of the middle ear muscles may attenuate the sound input by as much as 20 dB. Such powerful control will only be expected to occur for sound frequencies in the range where transmission is strongly affected by the middle ear muscle reflex, that is, below 1 kHz (Chapter 2). It will not explain the wide dynamic range of hearing for frequencies of 1 kHz and above.

9.5.1.5 The olivocochlear bundle

The olivocochlear bundle attenuates the responses of auditory nerve fibres by reducing the degree of active amplification of the travelling wave in the cochlea. Stimulation of the olivocochlear bundle can enhance the contrast in a spectral pattern for certain types of stimuli at high intensity and give a small increase in the upper limit of the dynamic range (Fig. 8.6B; Winslow and Sachs, 1987; Kawase et al., 1993). The mechanism was discussed in Chapter 8.

9.5.1.6 Conclusions

At high stimulus intensities, changes in psychophysical frequency resolution reflect the changes in the frequency resolution of the cochlea. However, the way that the auditory nerve transmits spectral information in this intensity range has not been definitively explained. Plausible hypotheses suggest that information in the time pattern of neural firings is used together with the information from small variations in mean firing rates (based on a range of thresholds in auditory nerve fibres, sloping saturations of the rate-intensity functions, and two-tone suppression). The middle ear muscle reflex and the olivocochlear bundle may also contribute.

9.5.2 Loudness

It has been suggested that the sensation of loudness depends on the total sum of activity transmitted in the auditory nerve (e.g. Wever, 1949). While this is likely to be true in general terms, it may not hold up in detail. The hypothesis moreover may not inform us about all the actual physiological mechanisms determining the sensation of loudness, which are likely to have a contribution from central processes.

Loudness can be assessed by asking the subject to adjust the levels of two stimuli so that one seems for instance twice as loud as the other. Clearly, this is a subjective judgement, and one amenable to many biases. The overall conclusion is that, for stimuli above about 40 dB SPL, a 10-dB increase in intensity generates approximately a doubling of loudness. Given that $\log_{10}(2)$ is approximately 0.3, this means that the amplitude of the loudness can be written as, Loudness $= k \times$ Intensity$^{0.3}$, where k is a constant.

This suggests that the activity generating the sensation of loudness is a compressive function of stimulus intensity.

In some ways, the growth of loudness mirrors the responses of the auditory periphery. As shown in Fig. 3.13A, above about 30 dB SPL, the amplitude of vibration on the basilar membrane grows non-linearly with stimulus intensity, with a compressive relation, and with a slope of about 0.3. Further stages of compression are the hair cell neural synapse, and all neural stages thereafter.

The growth of loudness mirrors other aspects of the response at the auditory periphery as well. Near threshold, and to a lesser extent at very high stimulus intensities, loudness grows more steeply with stimulus intensity (see, e.g., Moore et al., 1997, Fig. 12). Similarly, basilar membrane intensity functions grow more steeply at low stimulus intensities, that is, before the outer hair cells have started to saturate, and there is evidence from some researchers that it may start to grow more steeply again at very high intensities, when the passive component of basilar membrane vibration overtakes the saturating active component (see Chapter 3 and Fig. 5.24).

The concepts described above have been applied to a quantitative model, where the possible physiological correlates of each stage have been spelled out. After an initial compressive stage, corresponding to the non-linear growth of the basilar membrane, the stimulus is detected by multiple auditory nerve fibres (or in psychophysical terms, by multiple psychophysical filters), and the outputs of all the filters summed. The parameters of the model have been chosen so as to fit the empirical data most closely: the rate of growth of the amplitude on the basilar membrane has been chosen to be 0.2 dB/dB, rather than the value 0.3 dB/dB which is observed in many animal studies (see Chapter 3), because this generates a growth of loudness at the output of the model which increases as Intensity$^{0.3}$, in closest accordance with the psychophysical findings (Moore et al., 1997).

Other aspects of loudness judgements have a correlate in the responses in the auditory periphery. Zwicker et al. (1957) asked subjects to judge the overall loudness of a band of noise, of constant total power, but variable bandwidth. They found that when the band of noise was narrower than the equivalent bandwidth of one psychophysical filter, the judgement of loudness was independent of the bandwidth of the noise. However, if the noise was spread beyond one psychophysical filter, the loudness increased, even though the total power of the noise remained the same (Fig. 9.10A). This can be seen as another expression of the amplitude compression mentioned above, where a greater total response is produced by putting half the total energy into each of two channels, rather than concentrating it all on one channel.

Pickles (1983) imitated the paradigm in measuring the responses of single fibres of the guinea pig auditory nerve. Instead of measuring the responses of many fibres to a band centred on one frequency, the converse experiment was performed, of measuring the response of one fibre to bands of noise centred on many frequencies, and summing the results. The results have the advantage that between–fibre variability is eliminated and give results for an array of fibres each of which is identical to the fibre being stimulated. In this case, as with the experiment of Zwicker et al., the summed activity tended to remain constant for narrow stimulus bandwidths and increase for wider bandwidths, even though the total stimulus power remained the same. The curves followed the psychophysical results at least in the low and middle range of intensities (Fig. 9.10B).

Although the above model fits with the physiological data in general terms, it may not always agree quantitatively and in detail. Relkin and Doucet (1997) presented a method for measuring the total integrated activity of auditory nerve fibres, from measuring the gross potentials of the auditory nerve. They found that the total auditory nerve response grew with a slope that was about half that expected if loudness was proportional to the total activity in the auditory nerve.

Relkin and Doucet pointed out another problem. Although human beings are able to match the loudness of intense low–frequency tones to those of intense high–frequency tones, this is not always possible when considering the integrated activity of the auditory nerve. The reason is that intense low-frequency tones

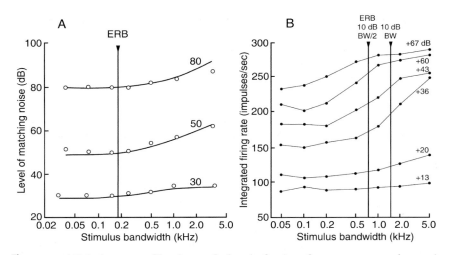

Fig. 9.10   (A) Judgement of loudness of a band of noise of constant power, but variable bandwidth. The band was matched in loudness to a 210-Hz wide band centred on the test frequency. The loudness stays approximately constant for bandwidths narrower than the width of a single psychophysical filter (ERB, arrowhead) and increases for wider bandwidths. ERB: equivalent rectangular bandwidth calculated for a psychophysical filter centred on the test frequency (1.42 kHz). Numbers on curves: total signal level in dB SPL. Solid lines: predictions from model of Moore *et al.* (1997). Data points from Zwicker *et al.* (1957). From Moore *et al.* (1997), Fig. 14. (B) Integrated firing rate of an auditory nerve fibre, as a function of stimulus bandwidth, for noise bands of constant total intensity. The integrated firing rate was calculated as described in the text. The numbers marked on the curves show the stimulus intensity, with respect to the fibre's absolute threshold. Near threshold, the integrated firing rate is relatively independent of stimulus bandwidth. At higher intensities, the integrated firing rate increases with stimulus bandwidth. The ERB of a fibre is expected to be about half the 10-dB bandwidth (arrowhead: 10-dB bandwidth, i.e. the bandwidth of the tuning curve measured 10 dB above the tip). Unlike in the original publication, a logarithmic scale of stimulus bandwidth is used, so that the results are more easily comparable with panel A. Fibre characteristic frequency: 3.76 kHz. Data from Pickles (1983), Fig. 2.

activate a large stretch of the basilar membrane, while intense high-frequency tones activate a much shorter stretch. This means that there are certain low-frequency tones which can never be matched in total activity by intense high-frequency tones, because the high-frequency tones can never generate enough total activity.

It is also highly likely that transformations of the auditory stimulus by the central nervous system play a critical part in determining the judged loudness of a stimulus.

Retro-cochlear tumours, such as vestibular schwannomas (also known as acoustic neuromas), that is, tumours that grow in the sheath of the vestibular nerve and affect hearing by pressing on the cochlear nerve and associated brainstem nuclei, can lead to an unusually slow growth in loudness, presumably because of decreased activity in the affected structures (e.g. Nieschalk *et al.*, 1999). This is in contrast to sensorineural hearing loss arising in the cochlea, which tends to lead to over-recruitment, that is, abnormally rapid growth of loudness with stimulus intensity (see Chapter 10).

9.6 SOUND LOCALIZATION AND SPATIAL HEARING

9.6.1 Introduction

A sound source in space will stimulate both ears. Experiments with headphones have suggested that the side on which a source is heard depends on timing and intensity differences at the two ears. A sound source on one side will stimulate the nearest ear first, because the sound path to that ear is shorter (Fig. 9.11A). This cue is particularly important for low frequency sounds, because with low frequency sounds, the phase differences at the two ears produced by the difference in path length are unambiguous. The intensity at the nearest ear will also be greater, because the farther ear is shadowed by the head. The degree of shadowing will be

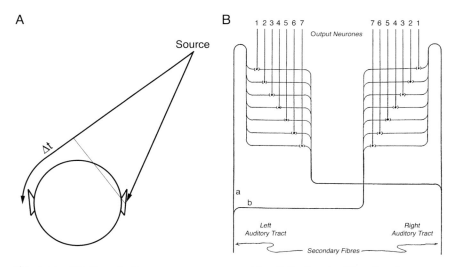

Fig. 9.11 (A) Sounds from a source to one side of the head will strike the nearer ear first (Δt: extra delay to farther ear) and will also be more intense in the nearer ear. (B) Jeffress's model of sound localization, based on neural delay lines. The output neurones marked '1' have the shortest neural paths from the ipsilateral side and the longest paths from the contralateral side. If the output neurones are driven by coincidence in their inputs, they will be activated when the difference in neural delays exactly compensates for the interaural delay Δt. Therefore, different output neurones will code different directions of the sound source. From Jeffress (1948), Fig. 1.

If however noise and tone were both presented simultaneously to the two ears, and the tone level was varied, the rate-intensity function to the tone could vary markedly with the phase of the tone. In some neurones, the masked response to the tone when it was presented in one phase could be an increase in activity, while in the opposite phase, the masked response could be a decrease in activity. In other neurones, tones always produced an increase in activity, but the rate-intensity function was shifted along the intensity axis. Differences in response as a function of phase, whether increases or decreases, can theoretically be used as a detection cue, and when the sizes of these cues are calculated over a population of neurones, BMLDs can be measured, although they are rather smaller than those found psychophysically in human beings (Palmer et al., 2000). Analogous results have also been found with more complex stimuli (Lane and Delgutte, 2005).

The mechanism behind the effect is likely to be the coincidence in activity from the two ears in driving the neurone, which then would be perturbed by the addition of a superimposed signal to one ear. Suppose a neurone as illustrated in Fig. 6.18A is stimulated with broadband noise, identical at the two ears, but with the contralateral ear leading by 200 μs. The neurone is driven by the coincidence of identical inputs from the two ears, which are in the optimal phase relation to give the maximal response. However, if a tone is superimposed on the input from one ear, the input waveforms from the two ears will no longer be identical. The phase difference between the waveforms from the two ears will vary from moment to moment because of summation of noise and tone in the input from one ear. Therefore, the stimuli from the two ears will no longer always be in an ideal phase relation to drive the neurone strongly. The firing rate of the neurone will therefore be lowered. In other neurones, with different relations between neurone characteristic frequency, tone frequency and characteristic delay, the effect of summation may be to increase the average firing rate.

The physiological data are in closest accordance with the model of interaural cross-correlation proposed by Colburn and Durlach (1978). In this model, the stimuli from each ear are initially narrowband filtered by a bank of filters, corresponding to the auditory nerve fibre filter functions. The inputs from the two ears are then cross-correlated within each frequency channel separately, so that the output signal from each channel is a function that plots the magnitude of the cross-correlation in that channel, as a function of all possible delays between the inputs from the two ears. Where the stimuli are identical at the two ears apart from being shifted in time, the function in any channel responding to the stimulus will have a single major peak. The value of the delay corresponding to the peak can be used to calculate the actual interaural delay, and hence the direction of the sound source at that frequency. The presence of stimuli which are different at the two ears will decorrelate the inputs and cause other, smaller peaks to appear in the functions, which can be used as a basis for detection (see e.g. Trahiotis et al., 2005).

An alternative model to explain the BMLD is the Equalization and Cancellation model. In this model, the activity from the two ears is subtracted, and the result is used to detect the signal (Durlach, 1972). Subtraction of the activity from the two ears can occur in the lateral superior olive (LSO). However, the LSO is mainly a high-frequency nucleus. One can speculate that the subtraction could instead occur in low-frequency cells of the LSO, if the LSO indeed has an inhibitory input in human beings, or it may be due to subtraction of the excitatory and the minority inhibitory inputs to the medial superior olive (see Section 9.6.2.2). However, physiological experiments with the stimuli that generate the BMLD, as described above, have not produced responses in accordance with this proposed mechanism.

The overall conclusion from the physiological studies is that the ability to hear sounds in a spatially complex auditory environment, known as spatial release from masking, uses mechanisms that are closely allied to those subserving sound localization and is based primarily on temporal cross-correlation occurring in the medial superior olive.

9.7 SPEECH

9.7.1 What is special about speech?

Speech is a highly practiced form of auditory perception. Speech sounds have many characteristics that are critical in the communication of meaning which mark them as different from other auditory stimuli and which carry the further implication that specialized neural structures have developed for the analysis of speech.

(i) As pointed out by Liberman et al. (1967), the individual perceived components of speech, that is, phonemes,[2] are not necessarily represented by individual sounds. Single acoustic cues often carry information simultaneously and in parallel about multiple phonemes, and information about single phonemes may be spread over successive acoustic cues. The acoustic cues used in identifying a single phoneme can vary enormously with the context and can depend on the sounds that come before or after. This permits the very rapid communication of meaning in speech and suggests that speech perception is based on learning patterns of speech on a larger scale than the phonemes, rather than by identifying the phonemes separately and in succession.

(ii) Speech sounds commonly show categorical perception. If one speech stimulus is manipulated so that it is gradually transformed to another speech stimulus, perception does not change gradually, but discontinuously (e.g. as when the sound 'ba' is transformed into the sound 'pa'). Moreover, thresholds for discrimination of differences well within one reported category are high, while thresholds for discrimination near the border between categories are much lower.

In speech, categorical perception is particularly seen in discriminating between phonemes based on their onsets (e.g. 'ba' vs. 'pa's above) and in discriminating between vowel sounds. While experiments measuring perception via conditioned reflexes show that very soon after birth newborn babies can discriminate well within single categories, and discriminate between the categories used in all languages equally well, by 12 months of age perception becomes dominated by the categories used in their native language. For instance, Japanese-learning babies lose

---

[2] Phonemes are defined as the smallest units of speech that change the meaning of a word if one is substituted for another.

the ability to discriminate 'la' and 'ra', which are both mapped to the same category in Japanese, while in English-learning babies the ability becomes enhanced (see Kuhl, 2004 for review). Some non-speech stimuli can also show categorical perception. It seems that categorical perception is valuable for the rapid and reliable detection and utilization of stimuli where identification of the category is critical, but discrimination within categories is not.

(iii) There are indications that listeners can switch between hearing some stimuli as speech or as non-speech, and that when they do, their ability to discriminate details of the stimuli change (for discussion of further evidence and for summary, see Moore, 2003).

(iv) Studies of brain function in human beings show that there are specialized regions for the analysis of speech. Observations from patients with lesions, and imaging the brain by functional magnetic resonance imaging (fMRI) or positron emission tomography (PET), suggest that some areas on the left hemisphere are more critical for the analysis of speech than of other stimuli. These findings will be discussed in more detail below.

In summary, many lines of psychophysical, anatomical, clinical and physiological data suggest that speech is at some stage analysed by specialized neural structures. It is quite possible that non-speech stimuli can also be analysed by these structures, and it is controversial as to what stage in the auditory pathway the structures become 'speech specific', if indeed they ever do. It is generally assumed, from the similarity of auditory anatomy in human and non-human species, that all structures up to and including the inferior colliculus and possibly the medial geniculate body deal with stimuli purely on the basis of their acoustic properties. To this extent, they are expected to deal equally with speech and non-speech stimuli. At some stage in cortical processing, structures are likely to become specialized for speech, and it is at the moment controversial whether this difference starts in the auditory core areas (e.g. AI) or develops only in higher order cortical areas (see discussion below).

It is therefore probably valid to analyse speech processing in the auditory brainstem by means of electrophysiological experiments in non-human species, using either human speech sounds or non-speech sounds that have been tailored to probe the mechanisms under consideration. However, at some level of the cortex, the mechanisms underlying the analysis of human speech can only be undertaken using speech stimuli in human beings. This means studies depend on functional imaging and anatomy in normal human beings and on data from, for example, lesions, microstimulation or neuronal multiunit and very occasionally single-unit recording, in clinical patients. Electrophysiological analyses of AI and other early cortical areas in animals have an uncertain status for the understanding of human processing of speech, with the interpretation of these experiments depending on the extent to which speech-specialized structures have developed in these areas in human beings. Some experimenters probe the responses of the cortex in non-human species with vocalizations specific to those species. This may give information on the mechanisms behind the responses to stimuli with speech-like levels of complexity, which are of critical importance for the species concerned.

To the extent that these underlying mechanisms may be common across species, the interpretation of the experiments may also be applicable to human beings.

9.7.2 Auditory nerve and brainstem responses

9.7.2.1 Vowel sounds

Given that the brainstem is likely to process speech sounds on the basis of their fundamental acoustic properties, analysis of speech sounds at this level can be undertaken with artificial speech-like stimuli in experimental animals. The coding of steady vowel sounds was studied by Sachs and Young (1979), who presented anaesthetized cats with steady-state synthesized vowel sounds, consisting of three formants, or spectral peaks, the lowest in frequency being called $F1$, the next $F2$ and the next $F3$. They used a limited set of vowels, and each was presented at several intensities. The activity of a large number of auditory nerve fibres was sampled in each animal in response to the same stimulus set. In this way, a picture was built up of the response of the whole nerve fibre array to each of the stimuli.

When mean firing rates were plotted as a function of fibre characteristic frequency, clear peaks at the frequencies of the formants could be seen in response to stimuli presented at low intensities (Fig. 9.13B). However, as the stimulus intensity was raised to 78 dB SPL and above, still in the range in which speech is easily comprehensible to human beings, the separate peaks disappeared, leaving a broad band of activation. The changes are most clearly shown in the graphs of the average responses at the bottom of the figure. Such a loss of spectral detail at medium and high stimulus intensities corresponds to that seen with other types of stimuli, when the responses of all fibres together are considered. The loss is due to three factors: (i) the flattening of the rate–intensity functions of the low-threshold fibres at high stimulus intensities, (ii) the reduction in cochlear frequency resolution expected at high stimulus intensities, and (iii) two-tone suppression, with the response to $F1$ suppressing the responses to $F2$ and $F3$. However, activity in those fibres tuned to frequencies in the gap between $F1$ and $F2$ is not suppressed: activity in these fibres is driven by $F1$ itself, and therefore is not suppressed by $F1$. Therefore, two-tone suppression reduces, rather than enhances, the spectral contrast in the responses of the nerve fibre array. However, and as with other types of stimuli, we expect the high-threshold fibres, which include those with sloping saturations or straight intensity functions, to convey some spectral details even at the higher stimulus levels (see Section 9.5.1.1 and Chapter 4).

In the cochlear nucleus, cells with excitatory tuning curves and inhibitory surrounds (Type II or III responses; Fig. 6.9) are able to represent spectral patterns in their mean firing rates over a wider range of stimulus intensities. Figure 9.13C shows the responses of sustained chopper cells in the cochlear nucleus, obtained by methods similar to those for the auditory nerve fibres in Fig. 9.13B. The peak of response to the lowest formant $F1$ is separate from the peaks to the two upper formants $F2$ and $F3$ at all stimulus intensities, although at the highest intensity, the peaks to $F2$ and $F3$ are not separable (see also averages at bottom of the figure). Sustained chopper cells are identified as T-stellate (T-multipolar) cells and have narrow tuning curves that are excitatory with inhibitory sidebands (Type III

9.7.2.2 Consonants

Transient speech sounds, such as consonants, produce temporally varying patterns of activity in different neurones, the pattern being determined by the time pattern of energy in the frequency channel to which the neurone is tuned.

In auditory nerve fibres, the patterns of firing can be predicted from the spectro-temporal pattern (spectrogram) of the speech sound and the frequency tuning of the fibres (Delgutte and Kiang, 1984b). At higher stimulus intensities in the auditory nerve, transient onset responses become relatively more prominent in the temporal pattern, probably because auditory nerve fibres have a greater dynamic range to transient than to steady-state stimuli.

In the cochlear nucleus and at higher levels, the responses of many neu-rones to frequency-modulated stimuli are enhanced. This emphasizes the responses to speech transients and to the temporal fluctuations in the speech waveform. Figure 9.14 compares sample responses from the auditory nerve, cochlear nucleus and inferior colliculus and shows how transients are particularly emphasized in the inferior colliculus. This forms an example of how certain critical features, in this case temporal transients and modulations, are progressively emphasized at higher and higher levels of the auditory system.

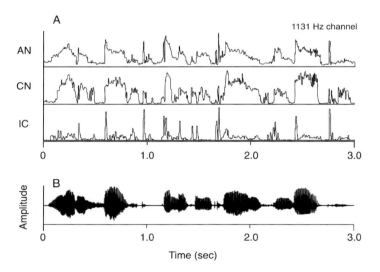

Fig. 9.14 (A) Responses of neurones in the auditory nerve (AN), cochlear nucleus (CN) and inferior colliculus (IC) to the speech sound 'wood is best for making toys and blocks' (waveform in B). Responses in the IC in particular show enhanced responses to the transients in the stimulus. For this figure, responses for neurones with characteristic frequencies within half an octave of 1131 Hz were averaged. The CN responses were recorded mainly from primary-like, chopper and pauser neurones. Data from Delgutte *et al.* (1998).

9.7.3 Cortical responses to vocalizations in non-human species

In an attempt to identify cortical mechanisms for the analysis of species–specific vocalizations, many experimenters have measured neuronal responses to specific, stereotyped animal vocalizations. For instance, Nagarajan *et al.* (2002) measured the responses of cells in the marmoset primary auditory cortex to a common call in the marmoset, the twitter call. When comparing different cells, the strength of response to the twitter calls could be related to the magnitude of the response to amplitude–modulated tones modulated at similar rates. The neurones appeared to be predominantly driven by the temporal properties of the stimulus, rather than by its spectral characteristics. Outside AI, the greater responsiveness to spectrally complex stimuli and to temporal modulation in many of the areas can be expected to further enhance the response to vocalisations (e.g. Tian *et al.*, 2001; Tian and Rauschecker, 2004; Gourevitch and Eggermont, 2007)

The overall conclusion from these and similar studies in animals has been that the responses of cortical neurones are determined by the general frequency and temporal properties of the sounds. So far, when considering the auditory core and belt areas in animals, there has been no evidence for specialized detectors of specific vocalizations. Rather, current models of coding suggest that the stimuli are represented as a pattern over a distributed neuronal population and use neuronal circuits that are shared with other auditory stimuli of similar complexity (see, e.g., Nagarajan *et al.*, 2002).

9.7.4 Responses to speech in the human cortex

9.7.4.1 The initial stage of speech processing in the human auditory cortex

Imaging studies in human beings show that both speech and non–speech stimuli activate areas on and around the superior temporal plane, which includes the auditory core areas (including AI in Heschl's gyrus) together with activation in other areas of the lateral surface of the brain (see Figs 7.4 and 9.16 for description of areas). The cortex is activated bilaterally, in the great majority of people to a greater extent on the left side (Fig. 9.15A). The extent of overall cortical activation varies between studies, being dependent on the type of task required by the subject in response to the speech (see, e.g., Martin, 2003 for review).

Figure 9.15B shows a detailed view of activation within the superior temporal plane, in a single slice 6 mm thick through the plane. The figure shows the response to words, when the subject had the task of distinguishing between words and 'pseudo–words', which were meaningless concatenations of syllables (Behne *et al.*, 2006). It shows how speech sounds bilaterally activate structures on the superior temporal plane. The stripes of activation visible in the image result from the gyri on the superior temporal plane moving in and out of the plane of section. In accordance with other studies, we also expect activation in many other areas, outside the section illustrated here.

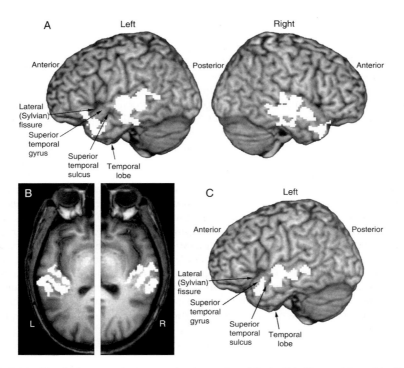

Fig. 9.15 Cortical responses to speech, shown in white in this Fig. and in red/yellow in Plate 6. (A) Response during passive listening to speech sounds, imaged in left and right hemispheres in a single subject by functional magnetic resonance imaging (fMRI). fMRI detects the local drop in oxygen level in the blood, consequent on activity. In this view, surface and subsurface signals from fMRI (coloured) are projected onto a standard cortical surface obtained from structural MRI. Areas (yellow/red) are shown where the signal with the speech sound is statistically greater than the signal in silence. Areas are bilaterally activated in the temporal lobe. Data for figure were provided by Professor C. Price. (B) Response to spoken words, imaged by fMRI in a 6-mm-thick slice along the surface of the superior temporal plane, in a single subject. The data from fMRI are superimposed on a high resolution structural MRI scan of the brain. There is a bilateral response, in Heschl's gyrus and extending over the superior temporal plane. The illustrated image is the average of the responses to the two ears and is the activity measured during presentation of the signal minus the activity measured in silence. Used with permission from Behne *et al.* (2006), Fig. 3, digital average of left halves of original sub-figures. (C) Responses to speech sounds, when the subjects had to make a later response based on the meaning of the sounds. The figure shows the activity in response to the speech sounds, minus the activity in response environmental sounds which were approximately matched in acoustic properties. There are discrete areas of specific activation in the region of the superior temporal gyrus and sulcus. Left hemisphere. Data from Thierry *et al.* (2003), as reanalysed by Price *et al.*, Reprinted from Price *et al.* (2005), Fig. 1A, Copyright 2005, with permission from Elsevier. See Plate 6.

At what stage in the cortex are speech stimuli analysed by speech-specific mechanisms, that is, where are speech stimuli treated differently from non-speech stimuli? This issue, which has been the object of many investigations over the years, is unfortunately an immensely difficult one to resolve. One of the problems is the difficulty of devising stimuli that are perceived as speech rather than as non-speech, while not differing in any other acoustic properties. Another difficulty is that any response to the speech may represent a high-level response to a semantic aspect of the stimulus, rather than the initial processing of the stimulus as speech.

For these reasons, different investigators have produced different results over the years. Figure 9.15C shows areas activated more by speech than by environmental sounds, as reported by Thierry et al. (2003). Analogous results have been found by others (e.g. Crinion et al., 2003; Liebenthal et al., 2005). The areas shown in Fig. 9.15C lie in the left middle and superior temporal gyri (Brodmann areas 21 and 22) and more anteriorly in the left temporal lobe (Brodmann area 38, near the temporal pole: see Fig. 9.16A for definition of areas). The areas lie within and just outside the cortical lateral parabelt areas (see Fig. 7.4). However, other investigators have pointed out that the stimuli used in such studies differ markedly in acoustic properties; a study where these were more closely controlled found only a single patch of potentially speech-specific activation in the centre of the areas shown in Fig. 9.15C (Uppenkamp et al., 2006). The results have the implication that the auditory core, belt and many parabelt areas, that is, the areas of the auditory cortex not highlighted in Fig. 9.15C, are involved in processing the general acoustic properties of all auditory stimuli, non-speech and speech stimuli alike.

These conclusions remain highly controversial; others using different paradigms find very different patterns of putative speech-specific activation (e.g. Whalen et al., 2006), and others dispute that the responses are indeed specific to speech (Price et al., 2005).

9.7.4.2 Higher levels of speech processing

Analysis of speech involves not only phonology, that is, the initial processing of speech sounds, but lexical analysis (analysis of words or groups of words), analysis of syntax (grammar) and semantics (meaning) (reviewed by Martin, 2003). Many of the relevant studies have used the production of speech or visual reading as tools. They are part of the large subject area of neurolinguistics and lie outside the scope of this book (see further reading at the end of this chapter).

A meta-analysis of a large number of imaging papers has suggested that structures on the left superior, middle and posterior temporal lobes are most closely associated with phonology (Vigneau et al., 2006). Also associated are areas in the left frontal cortex, around the posterior inferior frontal gyrus (parts of Brodmann's areas 44 and 45, previously known as Broca's area; for definitions of areas see Fig. 9.16A).

In the analysis suggested by Vigneau et al. (2006), information resulting from the phonological processing in the superior temporal plane is passed posteriorly to an area on the posterior superior temporal gyrus and sulcus for semantic processing.

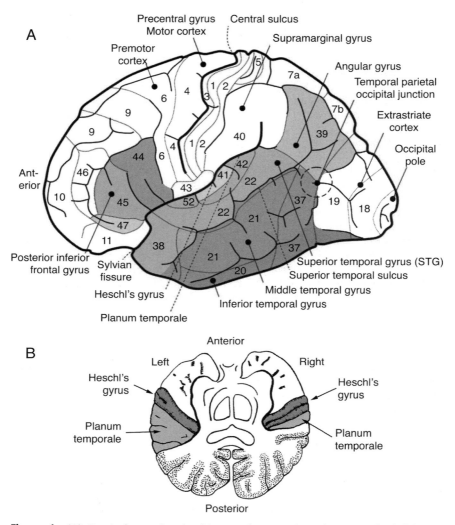

Fig. 9.16 (A) Cortical areas involved in speech processing, shown on the left hemisphere. Areas referred to in the text are shown coloured. Areas are numbered according to Brodmann (1909). Compare to Fig. 7.4 for more information. Solid lines indicate sulci, dotted lines the divisions between Brodmann areas. Used with permission from Démonet *et al.* (2005), Fig. 6. (B) Cortical asymmetry as reported by Geschwind and Levitsky. The figure shows an approximately horizontal section through the brain to reveal the upper surface of the superior temporal plane. The planum temporale is larger on the left side; the difference in this example is particularly dramatic. From Geschwind and Levitsky (1968), Fig. 1, reprinted with permission from AAAS. See Plate 7.

This area is activated for instance more by words rather than by pseudo-words (see, e.g., Okada and Hickok, 2006). The information is then processed syntactically in the posterior part of the superior temporal sulcus and then passed still more posteriorly to the angular gyrus for conceptual processing.

A second stream passes the information more anteriorly in the temporal lobe. The middle superior temporal gyrus includes an area that responds to the human voice and to speech sounds (the 'voice area') and shown as the central area of activation in Fig. 9.15C. An overlapping ventral part of this area is involved in semantic processing, that is, is more activated by intelligible words than by words that are spectrally modified so as to be unintelligible (e.g. Scott et al., 2000). A more anterior region of the temporal lobe, the temporal pole (junction of anterior Brodmann's areas 21 and 38) appears to be involved in the comprehension of sentences as well as in phonology.

In addition to the structures on the superior and anterior temporal lobe, the so-called language network incorporates the left posterior inferior temporal gyrus, the left angular gyrus and structures on the frontal lobe (including those previously known as Broca's area). On the right hemisphere, language processing involves the inferior temporal region and the right angular gyrus. The widespread participation of these structures may reflect the involvement of working memory as well as lexical and syntactic analysis (reviewed by Indefrey and Levelt, 2004 and by Vigneau et al., 2006). The involvement of the posterior inferior frontal gyrus and adjacent structures in the comprehension of language has been suggested to also result from their possible role in the sequencing of complex hierarchical or sequential structures.

Data from patients with lesions have, as commonly interpreted, pointed to two areas specifically involved in speech, previously known as Wernicke's and Broca's areas. Wernicke's area is now referred to as the posterior left superior temporal gyrus, that is, the most posterior part of Brodmann's area 22 (see Fig. 9.16A). Broca's area is now referred to as the left posterior inferior frontal gyrus, that is, parts of Brodmann's areas 44 and 45.

Lesions in the posterior left superior temporal gyrus give rise to problems in comprehension. While speech production may be grammatically normal, the resulting sentences can be meaningless, suggestive of the problems in comprehension. Imaging shows that this area has however multiple and diverse functions, being activated by a variety of events, including the perception of language-related sounds, monitoring the speakers own voice and the retrieval of words (for review, see Wise et al., 2001). Studies have found that lesions in this area do not in fact affect the comprehension of some sentences at all, although lesions in the middle temporal gyrus and anterior superior temporal gyrus can do so (reviewed by Dronkers et al., 2004). The latter areas on the temporal gyri are also the ones shown to be activated by speech in Fig. 9.15C. On the other hand, the left posterior inferior frontal gyrus is predominantly involved in the production of speech: lesions here leave comprehension relatively unaffected, although there can be problems in understanding long and syntactically complex sentences, commensurate with their potential role in processing complex hierarchical structures.

9.7.4.3 Left–right cortical asymmetries in auditory processing

Observations from brain lesions in human beings originally pointed to the importance of the left hemisphere for speech processing in the great majority (96%) of cases. Anatomical studies show that the superior temporal cortex usually has a larger surface area on the left than on the right side (Fig. 9.16B; Geschwind and Levitsky, 1968; see also Dorsaint-Pierre et al., 2006). The difference is particularly apparent in the planum temporale, which extends farther posteriorly on the left and which on average is one-third larger in area than on the right. The left planum temporale contains more white matter than the right, suggesting a greater extent of myelination, together with more interconnecting nerve fibres and a greater number of afferent fibres (Penhune et al., 1996). The left primary auditory cortex also contains larger pyramidal cells in layer III and wider cell columns (Seldon, 1981).

Observations in aphasic patients have for many years suggested that deficits in temporal processing underlie some of the language disturbances seen with left hemisphere lesions. Imaging studies using positron emission tomography show that tonal stimuli with many rapid temporal transitions activate the region around Heschl's gyrus to a greater degree on the left than on the right side (Zatorre and Belin, 2001). Recordings from human patients with electrodes placed within the auditory areas also have shown that stimuli with more temporal contrasts activated Heschl's gyrus and the planum temporale on the left more than the right side (Liegeois-Chauvel et al., 1999). The results did not apply only to speech sounds, but applied also to non-speech sounds with similar temporal structure. On the other hand, stimuli with slow temporal transitions preferentially activate the right hemisphere (Shtyrov et al., 2000). In addition, stimuli to the right ear have a small but significant advantage for the perception of speech. Because of the stronger crossed projection in the auditory system, we would expect these stimuli to preferentially activate the left hemisphere. The right ear advantage is particularly marked for stimuli with strong acoustic transients, such as consonants, whereas vowels which have slower temporal variations do not show a right ear advantage. This suggests that the left hemisphere is specialized for processing faster temporal variations than the right hemisphere. The higher degree of myelination of fibres in the left auditory areas would allow the more rapid local transfer of information, enhancing the processing of stimuli where timing is critical.

The asymmetry is carried through to complex syntactic function, as patients with left hemisphere lesions have more severe impairments in grammar and syntax than do patients with right hemisphere lesions. However, it appears that the right hemisphere preferentially, although not exclusively, processes the emotional content of words. For instance, patients with lesions of the parietal area of the right hemisphere are more impaired in the perception of the emotional content of speech than are those with lesions in the left hemisphere. However, patients with frontal lesions are equally impaired with lesions on either side (Shamay-Tsoory et al., 2004; Schirmer and Kotz, 2006).

9.8 Summary

1. The behavioural absolute threshold is related to the minimum thresholds of single auditory nerve fibres, determined from the mean firing rate.

2. The shape of the audiogram (the relation between threshold and stimulus frequency) is, for most of the audible frequency range, governed by the efficiency of the middle and outer ears in delivering energy to the cochlea. The cochlea itself has approximately equal sensitivity to energy of all frequencies, except at low (<450 Hz) and very high frequencies.

3. Frequency resolution describes the ability to filter out, on the basis of frequency, one stimulus component from another in a complex stimulus. Psychophysical frequency resolving power, as shown by 'psychophysical filters' or critical bands, seems to approximately match the frequency resolving power of the mechanical travelling wave in the cochlea and that of auditory nerve fibres. However, the correspondence varies with the psychophysical method used to measure the frequency resolution.

4. Because the cochlea behaves non-linearly, psychophysical methods using simultaneous masking, where the signal and masker have the opportunity to interact nonlinearly, give different results from those determined by non-simultaneous masking, for example, forward masking. In general, we expect psychophysical filters measured with simultaneous masking to be broader than those of the underlying physiological filters, especially on the high frequency side of the filters. Non-simultaneous masking techniques are expected to give more accurate measures of underlying physiological frequency resolution.

5. In pitch discrimination, two tones are presented successively, and we have to tell whether there is a difference between them on the basis of frequency. At high frequencies (above the frequency limit for phase locking, 5 kHz), it is likely that pitch discrimination takes place on the basis of differences in the place of activation along the cochlear duct. At lower frequencies, it is likely that temporal information is used. Neural recordings suggest that cells in the inferior colliculus are able to detect differences in the frequency of stimulation on the basis of timing information, at least for frequencies below 1 kHz. However, the underlying neural mechanisms are still controversial.

6. Psychophysical filters, and mechanical filtering functions on the basilar membrane, broaden with increases in stimulus intensity, and both do so in the same way. It is therefore very likely that the changes in frequency resolution with stimulus intensity at least partly reflect changes in cochlear filtering. Different nerve fibres have different thresholds and dynamic ranges. At high stimulus intensities, information reflecting mean firing rates is carried by a smaller subpopulation of fibres with high thresholds and wider dynamic ranges (those with 'sloping' and 'straight' saturations). In the cochlear nucleus and beyond, neurones with strong lateral inhibition are able to signal details of the stimulus in their mean firing rates over a wide range of stimulus intensities. Temporal information is preserved in the firing of auditory nerve fibres over the whole intensity range.

structures involved in temporal analysis, see Schirmer (2004). For reviews on imaging in relation to the aphasias and brain lesions, see Dronkers *et al.* (2004) and Lee *et al.* (2006), and in relation to the concept of Wernicke's area, see Wise *et al.* (2001). For a review of positron emission tomography in relation to auditory processing, see Ruytjens *et al.* (2006).

CHAPTER TEN

SENSORINEURAL HEARING LOSS

Hearing loss that arises in the cochlea, from damage to the hair cells or auditory nerve, is known as sensorineural hearing loss. Further cochlear losses can arise in the stria vascularis. In many cases, the causes of these losses are now known. In addition, sensorineural hearing loss has provided us with many models that have led to greater understanding of basic biological processes within the cochlea. The biological origin of the major forms of hearing loss will be discussed, and their correlates in terms of auditory performance will be described. The possibilities of reversing or restoring lost hearing by therapy at a cellular level, including stem cell therapy, gene therapy and antioxidant therapy, will be discussed, as will the restoration of hearing by cochlear prostheses. This chapter requires knowledge of Chapter 3 and the first part of Chapter 4.

10.1 TYPES OF HEARING LOSS

Hearing loss arising in the auditory periphery is divided into two types, known as conductive and sensorineural loss. Hearing loss due to an abnormality in the outer or middle ears is known as conductive loss. Conductive loss may arise for a number of reasons: the outer ear may be blocked or the tympanic membrane damaged, or the coupling of energy to the cochlea is reduced, because for instance the ossicles are immobilized, or because the differential transfer of pressure to the oval and round windows is otherwise impaired. Conductive loss produces a simple though frequency-dependent attenuation of the stimulus and can be well compensated for by hearing aids. In some cases, the causes are amenable to treatment by antibiotics, and in severe cases, the loss may be amenable to surgical intervention, for instance by a prosthesis replacing an ossified stapes in the oval window.

Hearing loss arising in the hair cells or auditory nerve is known as sensorineural hearing loss. Loss arising in the nerve sometimes results from a benign tumour around the sheath of the vestibular nerve (vestibular schwannoma, otherwise called an acoustic neuroma). However, the most common form of sensorineural impairment arises within the cochlea. The stria vascularis is a further vulnerable structure, giving a 'metabolic' or 'strial' type of loss. Cochlear hearing loss can also be caused by acoustic trauma, drugs, infections or may be congenital. A further common type of cochlear hearing loss arises in middle and old age, when degenerative changes can produce an impairment known as presbyacusis, which can be severe

10.2.1.2 Other ototoxic agents

Other agents will be mentioned only briefly. Cisplatin (cisplatinum), an anticancer compound that can cause permanent hearing loss, targets outer hair cells, cells of the spiral ganglion (auditory nerve) and the lateral wall of the cochlea, including the stria vascularis. It probably also works by oxidative damage, as antioxidants provide some protection (for review, see Rybak et al., 2007). Loop diuretics (e.g. ethacrynic acid, furosemide and bumetanide) reduce the absorption of fluid in the kidney by inhibiting the active absorption of Cl^- in the loop of Henle. In the cochlea, they affect the endocochlear potential, targeting the $Na^+/2Cl^-/K^+$ cotransporter in the marginal cells of the stria vascularis (Ikeda et al., 1997; see also Chapter 3). Aspirin (acetyl salicylate) causes a temporary hearing loss, by reversibly competing with Cl^- for a binding site on prestin, the outer hair cell motor protein that is responsible for the active amplification of the mechanical travelling wave in the cochlea (Santos-Sacchi et al., 2006). Salicylate induces tinnitus by mechanisms unknown; it does not increase spontaneous activity in the auditory nerve, but may act by central mechanisms (Muller et al., 2003; Wang et al., 2006). Organic solvents such as styrene and toluene are also ototoxic, although the mechanisms of the ototoxicity are not clear (Gagnaire and Langlais, 2005).

10.2.2 Acoustic trauma

Hair cells have been examined from cochleae either immediately after the induction of experimental acoustic trauma or after a period in which the degenerative or repair processes have had a chance to operate.

In the mildest cases of acoustic trauma, the stereocilia of outer hair cells can be slightly splayed and tip links broken, while the rootlets of the stereocilia become less dense in transmission electron micrographs (Liberman and Dodds, 1987; Clark and Pickles, 1996). It was suggested, on the basis of the losses in associated electrophysiological recordings, that these changes are fully reversible. In more severe cases, leading to permanent damage, the stereocilia kink or fracture at the rootlet and the packed actin filaments which give the stereocilia their rigidity depolymerize (Liberman and Dodds, 1987). The links between the stereocilia break and the stereocilia separate widely, with loss of tip links and consequent loss of transduction. In inner hair cells, however, the tallest stereocilia in the bundle tend to break away from the others, the shorter stereocilia keeping their linkages intact and hence presumably still being able to transduce (Fig. 10.3; Pickles et al., 1987b). In other cases, the stereocilia become fused, bent, splayed apart or detached (Fig. 10.4). In more severe cases, changes are also found in the supporting cells, and in very severe acoustic trauma, such a blast noise, the whole organ of Corti can be ripped apart mechanically (Patterson and Hamernik, 1997).

Intracellularly, hair cells show changes associated with metabolic stress, including breakdown of internal structures and swelling and disruption of mitochondria, which can be expected to lead to cell death over hours or days (Lim, 1986). As with otoxicity, oxidative damage may contribute to cell death, since enhanced

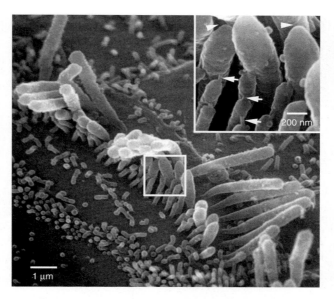

Fig. 10.3 The tallest stereocilia on an inner hair cell can show disarray after acoustic trauma, while the shorter stereocilia and their tip links remain intact. The inset shows the region outlined on the main figure and shows that tip links (arrows) remain on the shorter stereocilia. However, the tip links connecting the shorter stereocilia to the tallest stereocilia are broken (arrowheads). It is possible that the shorter stereocilia may still be moved by viscous drag from the surrounding fluid during acoustic stimulation. Scale bar: 1 μm on main figure and 200 nm on inset. Reprinted from Pickles *et al.* (1987b), Figs 15 and 16, Copyright (1987), with permission from Elsevier.

levels of reactive oxygen species can be demonstrated in hair cells after acoustic overstimulation (for review, see Henderson *et al.*, 2006). The reactive oxygen species are likely to have been produced by impaired oxidation in partially damaged mitochondria.

Further changes are produced in the afferent nerve supply. The synapses of the majority Type I afferent nerve fibres below the inner hair cells become swollen and can fragment. The changes are produced by excitotoxicity, that is, by the afferent neurotransmitter, glutamate, which activates channels in the nerve fibre membranes allowing high levels of Ca^{2+} to enter the cell. The Ca^{2+} has a number of effects: it activates many enzymes which damage cell structures such as the cytoskeleton, membranes and DNA as well as opening the permeability transition pores of mitochondria which can trigger cell death (see Box 10.2). In mild cases, the synapses can recover after a few days, but in more severe cases, the afferent nerve fibres degenerate. Anoxia can also cause excitotoxic damage to the afferent nerve fibres (for review, see Pujol and Puel, 1999).

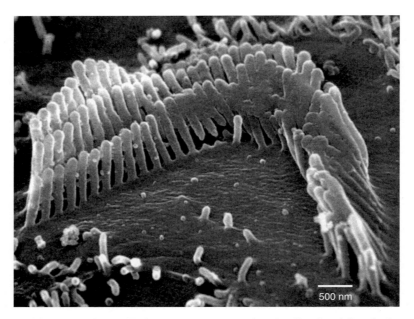

Fig. 10.4 An outer hair cell after acoustic trauma, showing fused and detached stereocilia and loss of tip links. Scale bar: 500 nm. Reprinted from Pickles *et al.* (1987b), Fig. 6, Copyright (1987), with permission from Elsevier.

10.2.3 Genetic causes

There are a large number of inherited diseases that can directly affect hearing. Many of these, though rare in the population as a whole, have been invaluable to researchers as a means of tracking down critical molecular components of the inner ear.

The most common genetic form of sensorineural deafness, in some national populations accounting for 35% of all cases of inherited hearing loss, is a mutation in the gene encoding connexin-26 (the *CX26* or *GJB2* gene), which gives rise to the form of deafness classed as DFNB1 (see Box 10.3). Connexin-26 is a component of gap junctions which allow ions and small molecules to pass between cells. In the inner ear, gap junctions in the supporting cells of the cochlea, in the spiral ligament and in the cochlear wall allow K^+ to be recycled from the scala tympani, through the spiral ligament, to the marginal cells of the stria vascularis, from where the K^+ is pumped into the scala media (see Chapter 3). DFNB1 is severe and of early onset. In gap junctions, connexin-26 can co-assemble with other connexins (e.g. connexin-30) to make a complete junction, and the gene for connexin-30 (*GJB6*) is sometimes also mutated, also giving rise to DFNB1 (for review, see Petersen and Willems, 2006).

Box 10.3   Nomenclature of genetic hearing losses

Genetic hearing losses are divided into Syndromic forms (where deafness is only one component of whole syndrome of changes, including, e.g., blindness), and Non-syndromic or Isolated forms (affecting hearing only).

Non-syndromic forms are further divided according to their mode of transmission:

(1) X chromosome–linked (labelled DFN).

(2) Y chromosome linked.

(3) Not linked to X or Y chromosomes (i.e. autosomal) and dominant (labelled DFNA).

(4) Not linked to X or Y chromosomes (i.e. autosomal) and recessive (labelled DFNB).

(5) Mitochondrial genes (maternally inherited).

Within the different categories, the type is labelled in order of date of identification, that is, DFNB1 was the first to be identified in the DFNB category. Human gene names are written in capitals, while other species have species-specific nomenclatures. In all species, gene names are written in italics, while gene protein products are written in non-italics.

Different mutations in the same gene can lead to different patterns of deficit (i.e. can give rise to different non-syndromic or syndromic losses).

From Petit (2006).

For example, among the many non-syndromic recessively inherited genetic diseases affecting hair cells, the first to be identified was one arising from mutations in the *MYO7A* gene. *MYO7A* codes for myosin 7A and gives rise to the DFNB2 hearing loss. Depending on the region mutated, mutations in *MYO7A* can also give rise to a syndromic hearing loss, Usher syndrome Type IB, which includes loss of vision as well as deafness. Myosin 7A is important for the integrity of the hair cell stereocilia. As a further example, the *CDH23* gene codes for cadherin-23 (otocadherin), a major component of the tip link, loss of which leads not only to loss of transduction, but to gross disorganization of the stereocilia and to the DFNB12 type of hearing loss. Thirdly, the *USH1C* gene was found to code for a cytoskeletal protein called harmonin, which is expressed in stereocilia and which cooperates with myosin 7A and cadherin-23 in generating the hair cell bundle (Boeda *et al.*, 2002). While mutations in this gene can give rise to the non-syndromic hearing loss labelled DFNB18, the pattern of mutations more commonly lead to Usher Syndrome Type 1C, which includes blindness as well as deafness. Many further genes also affect hair cells and also give rise to deafness when mutated: for reviews, see Petersen and Willems (2006) and Petit (2006).

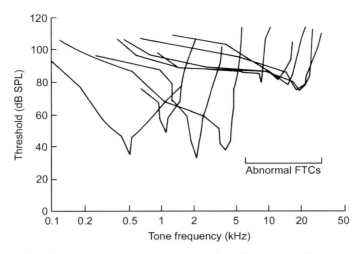

Fig. 10.5   After kanamycin, the tuning curves of auditory nerve fibres are raised in threshold and broadened in shape. In this experiment, fibres from the high-frequency end of the cochlea were most affected ('Abnormal FTCs'). Guinea pig. From Evans and Harrison (1976), Fig. 1.

broadened in shape (Fig. 10.6A; Liberman and Dodds, 1984b). If however some outer hair cell stereocilia remained, a small, sharply tuned tip could remain on the upper edge of the tuning curves, presumably resulting from only a partial loss of the sharply tuned response (Fig. 10.6B). These results confirm the role of the outer hair cells in increasing the sharp tuning and sensitivity of the travelling wave.

10.3.1.2 Damage to inner hair cells

The majority of experimental manipulations affect outer hair cells rather than inner hair cells. However, by tracing horseradish peroxidase-filled afferents to the inner hair cells after electrophysiological recordings, Liberman and Dodds (1984b) were able to show that where there was disarray mainly of inner hair cell stereocilia, the tuning curves were raised in threshold, but were of nearly normal shape (Fig. 10.6C). The results are in agreement with the idea that inner hair cells are only involved in detecting the movement of the basilar membrane and are not involved in producing the sharp tuning. The disarray was mainly seen in the tallest stereocilia; the morphological changes shown in Fig. 10.3, where the tip links remain intact on the shorter stereocilia, suggest that such inner hair cells might indeed be able to continue transducing, though with reduced sensitivity. Auditory nerve fibres from these inner hair cells have much lowered rates of spontaneous activity, perhaps because of reduced standing currents through the disconnected, and therefore possibly shut, mechanotransducer channels (Liberman and Dodds, 1984a).

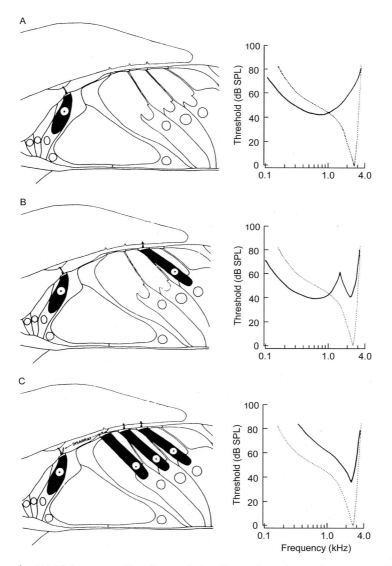

Fig. 10.6 (A) If the stereocilia of outer hair cells are lost, the auditory nerve fibres innervating the adjacent inner hair cells are raised in threshold and broadened in tuning (solid line in tuning curve vs. dotted line – normal). The low-frequency tail of the tuning curve becomes hypersensitive. (B) If some outer hair cell stereocilia remain, a short, sharply tuned tip can be seen on the tuning curve. (C) If inner hair cell stereocilia are damaged while most outer hair cell stereocilia remain apparently normal, the tuning curve can have a nearly normal shape but be raised in threshold. Reprinted from Liberman and Dodds (1984b), Fig. 14, Copyright (1984), with permission from Elsevier.

10.3.2 Psychophysical correlates
10.3.2.1 Threshold and loudness

The neural data lead us to expect a loss of sensitivity in sensorineural hearing loss of cochlear origin, combined with a loss in frequency resolution.

The loss of sensitivity is of course an easily recognizable sign of cochlear damage. In ototoxicity and ageing, high frequencies are generally affected first, in accordance with the generally greater vulnerability of basal outer hair cells (see Section 10.2). However, with acoustic trauma, the losses are determined by the frequency of exposure as well as by the pattern of vulnerability of the hair cells.

With intense narrowband traumatizing stimuli, it can be shown that the losses are concentrated at the point of maximum vibration of the basilar membrane, which leads to a loss of sensitivity to frequencies represented in that region. However, it should be noted that the frequency of maximum loss and the frequency of exposure are not always the same. As shown in Fig. 3.10B, with intense stimuli the peak of mechanical vibration occurs basal to the peak measured with less intense stimuli (compare lines for 100 dB SPL and 20 dB SPL). This occurs because the peak of vibration for less intense stimuli is dominated by the active process. The active process starts to grow more slowly beyond around 30 dB SPL. However, the passive component of the travelling wave, though smaller at low-stimulus intensities, increases linearly with intensity, and so comes to dominate at high stimulus intensities. The peak of vibration for the 15 kHz 100 dB SPL stimulus in Fig. 3.10B, at around 3.1 mm from the base, corresponds to the 18 kHz point in the cochlea, if measured with low–intensity test stimuli. In this example, intense 15-kHz tones will therefore produce their greatest losses at around 18 kHz. The phenomenon, of intense narrowband stimuli producing maximum losses in sensitivity at higher frequencies, is known as 'the half–octave shift'. The same phenomenon is depicted in Fig. 8.5, where a 10-kHz traumatizing tone produces the greatest threshold loss at 14 kHz.

In human beings, general broadband noise exposure, as found for instance in a noisy environment, commonly produces its first loss at 4 kHz, producing a phenomenon in the audiogram known as the '4 kHz notch'. A selective loss at this frequency is generally taken as a sign of previous noise exposure, though with limited reliability (see, e.g., McBride and Williams, 2001). The mechanisms behind the development of the 4-kHz notch are not known. It may correspond to a particular vulnerability of the cochlea in this region, combined with the overall spectrum of the noise to which individuals tend to be exposed. A 4-kHz notch is also seen in the behavioural audiograms of apparently normal cats, and in the thresholds of auditory nerve fibres with characteristic frequencies in that region (Fig. 4.5). These small losses in apparently normal cats seem to be pathological, because they are reduced in cats raised from birth in a soundproofed chamber (Liberman and Kiang, 1978).

Patients with sensorineural hearing loss show a characteristic feature, namely that of loudness recruitment. Once stimuli become suprathreshold, perceived loudness grows abnormally quickly with increases in stimulus intensity. Originally, it was thought that this had a cochlear origin and could be explained by the transition from the generally shallow slope of the amplitude functions that are seen in sensitive cochleae, to the steeper more linear growth seen in insensitive cochleae (see, e.g., Fig. 3.13A, compare curves marked 9, 10 and 11 kHz with that marked 9 pm). However, recordings from auditory nerve fibres are inconsistent with this hypothesis: loudness functions calculated from the responses of auditory nerve fibres are no steeper after hearing loss than before (Heinz *et al.*, 2005). It was postulated that recruitment, instead, arose from a central hypersensitivity to auditory stimuli following peripheral hearing loss.

10.3.2.2 Frequency resolution

The change in neural frequency resolution similarly has a correlate in psychophysical data. Psychophysical turning curves, which are thought to be an approximation to neural turning curves (Fig. 9.4), are broadened (e.g. Moore and Glasberg, 1986). The sharply tuned tip of the psychophysical tuning curve is shortened or abolished, and the low-frequency slope in particular becomes shallower (Fig. 10.7). These changes parallel those seen in auditory nerve fibres (Fig. 10.5). In some cases, W-shaped FTCs are found. These do not have an obvious correlate in the tuning curves of auditory nerve fibres. Instead, Kluk and Moore (2005) showed that W-shaped tuning curves in impaired ears occurred when the signal frequency fell within or near a cochlear 'dead' region, that is, one in which no responses were detectable because for instance none of the inner hair cells is functional. In these cases, the signal was detected in other frequency regions of the cochlea, as a result of beats or difference tones produced between the signal and the masker.

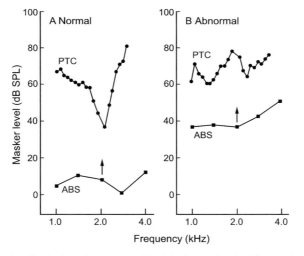

Fig. 10.7 Psychophysical tuning curves (PTCs) determined with simultaneous masking in a normal subject (A) and in a subject with sensorineural hearing loss (B). ABS: absolute threshold (audiogram). Arrows: frequency and intensity of probe. Reprinted from Carney and Nelson (1980), Figs 1 and 3, Copyright (1983), with permission from American Institute of Physics.

Additional masking of these components returned the FTCs to a simple shape, with a single broad dip.

Critical bandwidths, being the bandwidths of the psychophysical filter (see Section 9.3.1.3), are also affected. Psychophysical filters, measured by a great variety of methods, all become broader with increases in threshold. For instance, Laroche *et al.* (1992) asked subjects to detect a probe tone masked by wideband noise, where the noise had a notch in its spectrum centred on the frequency of the probe. They plotted the masked threshold as a function of the width of the notch and used the results to calculate the shape of the psychophysical filter. There was little change in the effective bandwidth of the psychophysical filter with threshold losses of up to about 30 dB, and thereafter bandwidths increased approximately 1.5-fold for each 10 dB increase in threshold. The same trend was apparent in a summary of data published by Moore (2005). These patterns of change have a parallel in the single unit data where for small losses the tips of the tuning curves are raised but do not become any broader, but after a certain point, the tuning curves broaden substantially.

There is also a very large scatter in the psychophysical data, some patients with hearing losses of up to 70 dB showing normal frequency resolution bandwidths. This may reflect variation in the factors underlying the loss (e.g. the relative degrees of damage to inner and outer hair cells).

The loss of resolution leads to a particular difficulty in understanding broadband complex sounds. While acoustic amplifying hearing aids can increase the magnitude of the acoustic signal, and so restore sensitivity, they cannot restore the cochlea's frequency resolution, so that the sounds, though now audible, may sound incomprehensible or garbled. This particularly affects the understanding of speech, especially in a noisy background.

10.3.2.3 Tinnitus

One of the sometimes distressing accompaniments of sensorineural hearing loss is tinnitus, which can deprive the sufferers of even the dubious consolation of living in a silent world. Tinnitus is defined as an auditory sensation in the absence of an auditory input. Originally, tinnitus was divided into objective tinnitus, which could be recordable as a real sound in the ear, and subjective tinnitus, which could not. Objective tinnitus was thought to arise peripheral to the cochlea, in say the muscles or vasculature of the middle ear, while subjective tinnitus arose in the cochlea or more centrally. The discovery of cochlear emissions showed that some 'objective' tinnitus could arise in the cochlea. Figure 5.20A shows a recording of spontaneous objective tinnitus of cochlear origin, recorded in the ear canal. It is likely that this arises when the gain of the outer hair cell active process becomes temporarily high, enhancing the energy fed back into the basilar membrane. If the spatial relations are right, mechanical energy may be reflected back and forth along the cochlea, further stimulating the hair cells, leading to a self-sustaining oscillation, and so to tinnitus. It is common to experience transient periods of tinnitus of this type, when a sudden tonal 'ping' is heard in the ear, which then gradually fades over several seconds or minutes. In these cases, an emission of sound of the same frequency can be recorded in the ear canal.

Although this is an intriguing explanation of one type of tinnitus, it is not likely to explain the majority of the cases of clinical importance. We expect tinnitus associated with cochlear emissions to be continuous and narrowband or tonal. In contrast, much tinnitus is continuous and atonal, like high pitched hissing or knocking noises. Moreover, cochlear emissions disappear in experimental cochlear deafness, while tinnitus can be particularly prominent in patients with severe hearing loss.

In contrast, most of the tinnitus of clinical importance is likely to arise centrally. This is supported by findings that cutting the auditory nerve is commonly ineffective in relieving tinnitus. Since tinnitus is usually associated with some degree of hearing loss, the most reasonable explanation is that tinnitus results from central hypersensitivity following a reduction in peripheral input.

Animal models have proved invaluable for analysing possible neural mechanisms for the generation of tinnitus. In a typical behavioural test, animals are trained to drink in the presence of noise, but trained to stop drinking when in silence (Jastreboff et al., 1988). Before the induction of tinnitus, animals are tested in alternating periods of noise and silence. After the experimental manipulation, continued drinking in the periods of silence is taken as an indication that the animals can in fact hear a stimulus, that is, can hear tinnitus. Factors that induce tinnitus when tested this way are similar to those inducing tinnitus in human beings, including systemically administered ototoxic drugs (aminoglycosides, salicylate and quinine) and acoustic overstimulation.

The tinnitus-inducing manipulations do not in general produce sustained increases in the spontaneous activity of primary auditory nerve fibres; rather, the activity decreases or stays the same (e.g. Mulheran, 1999). However, spontaneous activity may increase in certain central structures of the auditory pathway, including the dorsal cochlear nucleus, the external nucleus of the inferior colliculus and areas of the auditory cortex (AI and AII). In contrast, the central nucleus of the inferior colliculus is not affected (for review, see Eggermont, 2005). It appears that, therefore, in the brainstem, the areas that are affected belong to the non-specific or extralemniscal auditory system surrounding the more specific auditory nuclei, with the dorsal cochlear nucleus potentially marking the first appearance of the extralemniscal pathway (see Chapter 6).

As an example, Kaltenbach et al. (1998) exposed hamsters to an intense (125–130 dB SPL) 10-kHz tone for 4 h. Thirty days after the exposure, rates of spontaneous activity were found to be raised three- to four-fold in the dorsal cochlear nucleus. Neural thresholds were also raised, consistent with the suggestion that increased thresholds can lead to increased spontaneous activity. Analogous effects have been seen with the ototoxic drug Cisplatin, the degree of increase in spontaneous activity being correlated with the degree of loss of the outer hair cells (Kaltenbach et al., 2002). GABA is a major inhibitory neurotransmitter within the DCN, and 30 days after acoustic overstimulation, levels of glutamate decarboxylase, one of its synthetic enzymes, were found to be lowered. This would decrease the availability of GABA and therefore reduce the amount of inhibition in the nucleus. The reduction in GABA levels can be reversed by the anti-epileptic drug vigabatrin, which inhibits one of GABA's degradative enzymes and so increases GABA levels. In experimental animals, vigabatrin was found to eliminate tinnitus, as judged by a behavioural test similar to the one described above (Brozoski *et al.*, 2007). Changes in GABAergic inhibition could also explain the increased tinnitus commonly found with ageing, since GABA is reduced in the auditory brainstem of ageing rats (Caspary *et al.*, 1995).

One of the critical features of tinnitus is the way that it can dominate the patient's attention. This can occur even though the tinnitus may be perceived at only a low subjective level, as judged by comparisons of loudness. It is noteworthy that the nuclei of the extralemniscal auditory pathway, where the enhanced activity has been shown with tinnitus-inducing stimuli, trigger automatic orienting reflexes, which may explain the effect (see Chapter 6). A further common finding is that tinnitus is enhanced by anxiety. Activity of the locus coeruleus induces anxiety, and the locus coeruleus sends projections to the dorsal cochlear nucleus (Kromer and Moore, 1980; Tanaka *et al.*, 2000). Cross-sensory interactions in tinnitus may also be explicable: in some patients, tinnitus can be enhanced by clenching the jaws or contracting muscles of the neck. Stimulation of the trigeminal and other somatosensory nerves can enhance responses in auditory neurones situated in the dorsal cochlear nucleus and external nucleus of the inferior colliculus, sites in the extralemniscal auditory pathway where neuronal activity is increased in tinnitus (Shore and Zhou, 2006; for review, see Kaltenbach, 2006).

Notwithstanding the preliminary results described above, tinnitus in human beings is currently poorly controlled by drugs or by surgery. However, behavioural intervention, in the form known as tinnitus retraining therapy, can be highly successful. Tinnitus retraining therapy aims to reduce the perception of tinnitus by reducing its significance for the patient. In this way, it is hoped that the mechanisms of neural plasticity that have enhanced the tinnitus in the patient's awareness will be put into reverse. Tinnitus retraining therapy uses multiple strategies, including counselling and the use of distracting sounds, to bring this about, with a reported success rate of 80% or higher (Jastreboff and Jastreboff, 2006).

10.4 PHYSIOLOGICAL ASPECTS OF THE COCHLEAR PROSTHESIS

10.4.1 Introduction

When the hair cells of the cochlea are lost in human beings, they cannot currently be replaced. Therefore, natural hearing cannot be restored. Under these circumstances, the best hope for restoring some auditory function seems to be to bypass the transducer mechanism and to attempt to stimulate what remains of the auditory nerve directly, by electrical means. It is intended, by stimulating early in the auditory pathway, that the complex and specialized signal processing capabilities of the auditory system will be utilized. Cochlear implants have been highly successful, restoring useful hearing at the time or writing to over 100,000 people worldwide. The successful development of effective cochlear prostheses has depended on the simultaneous solution to problems in physiology, bioengineering, psychophysics and signal processing.

The earliest attempts to stimulate the cochlea by means of a prosthesis ranged from the use of a single extracochlear electrode on the round window to intra-cochlear stimulation with one or a few electrodes. These devices generally gave poor sound quality, and unaided speech perception was rarely attainable. Development of an effective prosthesis, with free-running conversational speech being understood by a high proportion of patients, has depended on (i) the development of longer electrode arrays, so that a greater length of the cochlea can be stimulated; (ii) the use of multiple electrodes, so that the stimulus could be delivered to local-ized regions of the cochlea; (iii) the development of novel patterns of electrical stimulation and advanced signal pre-processing, which present the cues to the remaining auditory nerve fibres in the most effective manner and (iv) advances in electrode design which have permitted the electrodes to be inserted accurately in the correct places in the cochlea while causing minimal damage and tissue reaction.

10.4.2 Physiological background
10.4.2.1 Condition of the nerve

A critical question is: are there any auditory nerve fibres left to stimulate when all hearing has been lost through cochlear deafness? In a summary of seven studies in human beings, Leake and Rebscher (2004) reported that the mean survival of cochlear ganglion cells varied between 41 and 77% of normal (range of averages for the different studies). The extent of the loss depends on the original cause of the deafness. There were large losses if the original deafness was due to viral labyrinthitis, fewer losses if it was due to congenital deafness or to bacterial menin-gitis, and only small losses if the original deafness was due to aminoglycosides or to sudden idiopathic deafness. In addition, the losses tended to be greater towards the base of the cochlea where most cochlear prostheses are placed, and the losses increased with longer durations of deafness (Nadol, 1997; see also Shepherd et al., 2004, for animal studies). However, it is difficult to assess this ahead of implan-tation: pre-operative testing for the presence of nerve fibres with, for example, extracochlear electrical stimulation has been shown to have limited predictive value and is therefore normally not undertaken (e.g. Frohne et al., 1997).

A second problem is that intracochlear insertion of the electrode array may produce further loss of nerve fibres. The major factor causing this arises from trauma during insertion, which may extend to the array breaking through the spiral lamina or through the covering of Rosenthal's canal, the latter containing the cells of the cochlear ganglion. A further complication is the growth of new bone around the electrode, which is probably determined both by the previous pathology and by the degree of trauma occurring during the insertion (Nadol, 1997).

10.4.2.2 Responses of auditory nerve fibres to electrical stimulation

In normal subjects, the auditory nerve transmits information by two methods of coding, namely (i) the place principle, by which the place of maximum activation in the cochlear duct depends on the frequency of the stimulus and (ii) the timing principle, by which individual action potentials tend to be locked to the temporal waveform of the stimulus. With normal acoustic stimulation, these are not independent factors, but are tied together by the mechanics of the cochlea. Furthermore at any one frequency, the firing rate increases sigmoidally with the stimulus intensity. It is worth examining the extent to which these aspects can be reproduced by electrical stimulation.

10.4.2.2.1 The place principle. If auditory nerve fibres are stimulated electrically, nerve fibres are seen not to have any intrinsic tuning at all. In the experiment illustrated in Fig. 10.8A, the cats were first deafened with an ototoxic antibiotic, so that there was no chance that the electrical stimulus would trigger a normal travelling wave. The electrical stimulus was applied to the round window. Irrespective of the fibre's place of origin along the cochlear duct, the lowest thresholds were produced with stimulus frequencies of around 100–200 Hz, and there was a gradual rise in thresholds towards higher frequencies of stimulation.

Analogous results have since been found by many other investigators (e.g. van den Honert and Stypulkowski, 1984). Therefore, if frequency information is to be transmitted as place information in the auditory nerve, ways must be found to restrict the stimulus to local regions of the cochlea. Current spread in the cochlea makes localized stimulation difficult. With monopolar stimulation, the current is applied to one electrode in the cochlear duct and flows to a remote electrode. With this configuration, there is a wide pattern of activation in the cochlear duct. In bipolar stimulation, currents flow between members of a pair of closely spaced electrodes, both of which are within the cochlear duct. Bipolar stimulation produces much more confined pattern of activation along the duct (van den Honert and Stypulkowski, 1987). However, and surprisingly, bipolar stimulation does not generally improve perception through the implant and therefore it is not usually used. A further reason for not using bipolar stimulation is that it needs much higher currents, by an order of magnitude or so, which results in significantly greater power consumption.

10.4.2.2.2 The timing principle. Temporal information is preserved with electrical stimulation. Indeed, firing tends to be restricted more closely to one point on the waveform than with acoustic stimulation, as shown in response to sinusoidal stimulation in Fig. 10.8B. This presumably occurs because as soon as the electric potential has reached the threshold for activation, the nerve fibre fires with a high probability. Figure 10.8C shows the precise timing of action potentials to the bipolar pulsatile stimuli as used in current implants. Although with electrical stimuli the maximum firing rates of auditory nerve fibres are in the range 800–1000/sec (e.g. Shepherd and Javel, 1997), some degree of phase-locking can be detected with much higher frequencies of stimulation (e.g. to 2.5 kHz; Parkins, 1989).

10.4.2.2.3 Rate-intensity functions. Figure 10.8D shows that rate-intensity functions to electrical stimulation are very steep indeed; that is, as with the time-varying stimuli discussed in Section 10.4.2.2.2, once threshold is reached, the

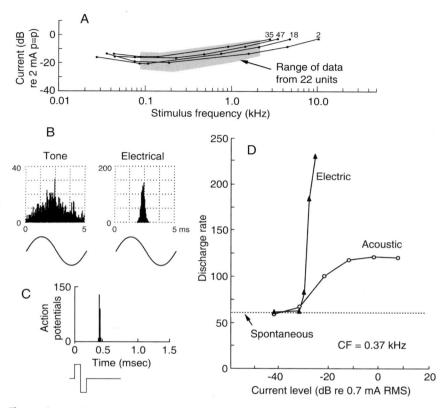

Fig. 10.8 Auditory nerve responses to electrical stimulation. (A) Auditory nerve fibres show negligible intrinsic tuning to electrical stimuli applied across the cochlea. These broad 'tuning curves' should be compared to the sharp tuning curves to acoustic stimuli shown in Fig. 4.4. (B) Period histogram in response to a 200 Hz sinusoidal acoustic stimulus in a normal cat (left) and of a sinusoidal electric stimulus in a deafened cat (right). With electrical stimulation, the actions potentials are triggered in a highly restricted region of the waveform. (C) Response to biphasic pulsatile stimulation, as currently used by cochlear implants. The latency of the response (depending on the neural travel time to the recording site) is approximately 0.5 ms. (D) The steep rate-intensity functions seen with electrical stimuli in an ototoxically deafened cat, compared with the shallower function found with acoustic stimuli in a normal cat. A, B and D from Kiang and Moxon (1972), Figs 1, 2 and 3; C reprinted from Javel and Shepherd (2000), Fig. 4, Copyright (2000), with permission from Elsevier.

fibre fires with a high degree of probability. The dynamic range is often less than 10 dB. This can be compared with 20–30 dB for low-threshold fibres, and 60 dB for high-threshold fibres, to acoustic stimulation. Moreover, the spread of thresholds in different fibres is very small, being less than 20 dB (van den Honert and Stypulkowski, 1987). This means that the spread of activity to extra fibres can provide only a very small extension of the dynamic range. The results mean that very accurate amplitude compression of the stimulus is necessary.

10.4.2.3 Insertion and pattern of stimulation

Modern multi-channel cochlear implants contain a pre-formed set of electrodes (between 6 and 22 in current devices) fixed in the surface of a long, tapered, silicone carrier. The cochlear wall is opened near the round window, and the electrode array is inserted into the scala tympani, to a maximum depth of between 20 and 25 mm. Because cells of the spiral ganglion are concentrated towards the base of the cochlea, insertion to this depth may cover a significant extent of the ganglion (Sridhar *et al.*, 2006). The implant can be preformed with a curve, so that after insertion, it hugs the inner, modiolar wall of the scala tympani as much as possible, with the result that the electrodes come to lie as close as possible to the cell bodies of the spiral ganglion ensuring low thresholds and a wider dynamic range (Shepherd *et al.*, 1993).

It has been found best to use brief (e.g. 25 μs) current pulses for stimulation. The pulses are delivered in a charge-balanced configuration, so that in one electrode a pulse of one polarity is followed by a second pulse of opposite polarity (Fig. 10.9). This means that during stimulation, there is ideally no net current flow through an electrode, so that any ionic changes produced during the first pulse

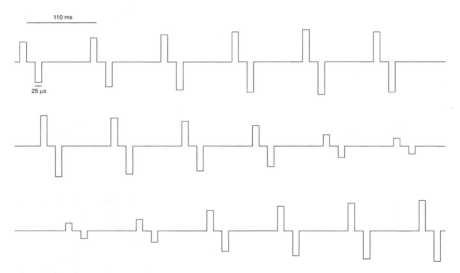

Fig. 10.9   The pattern of electrical stimulation commonly used in a cochlear implant, illustrated for three electrodes. Brief charge-balanced pulses (10–50 μs each) are presented at a rate of between 200 Hz and 2 kHz per channel (900 Hz illustrated here). The amplitude of stimulation is varied independently at each electrode. The different channels are activated at different times to reduce current flow between channels.

should be exactly reversed during the second pulse. Pulses are delivered asynchronously to the different channels in the implant, to reduce electrical interaction between the different channels. Each channel is stimulated at a rate of between 200 and 2000 pulses/sec. For most patients, the electrodes are driven in a monopolar configuration, that is, with current applied between the active scala tympani electrode and a remote ground, which is typically an electrode on the implanted receiver–stimulator or located in the temporalis muscle. However, many devices are reprogrammable, so that bipolar stimulation or 'common ground' stimulation (where all the inactive electrodes can be used as a ground for the electrode in use) can also be used. Modern cochlear implants also include an option for telemetry, with signals being transmittable in reverse from the device to an external receiver, so that the patient's neural responses to stimulation can be measured by the clinician. This facility can also measure the impedance of each electrode.

10.4.3 Results

10.4.3.1 Intensity coding

As expected from the physiological experiments, the dynamic range, being the range between threshold and discomfort, is small. Dynamic ranges are commonly around 10 dB, though much smaller and much larger values can be found (e.g. Zeng and Shannon, 1994; Nelson *et al.*, 1996). The dynamic range can be markedly different between electrodes in a single patient. It might be thought that if the stimulus were more localized in the cochlea by using for instance bipolar stimulation, increased current spread with intensity might increase the dynamic range. However, this does not appear to be the case (e.g. Cohen *et al.*, 2001). The narrow dynamic range, presumably associated with a steep dependence of loudness on stimulus intensity, does not seem to have correlate in particularly small difference limens for intensity. Difference limens are about 1 dB, similar to those found with acoustic stimuli. Over the whole dynamic range, therefore, there may be only about 10–20 just noticeable difference for intensity, although with enormous variations between subjects and electrodes, compared with well over 100 for normal hearing.

10.4.3.2 Frequency, pitch and stimulus quality

If we believe the extreme position that at low frequencies information is carried purely by the temporal pattern of nerve impulses, then periodic electrical stimulation should produce faithful representation of auditory sensations and good discrimination of frequencies. The results of electrical stimulation have been disappointing for such a prediction. In only a few cases do electrical stimuli produce clear tonal sensations. A typical report is that tones sound harsh or like a buzz.

Nevertheless, a subjective pitch can often be ascribed to the stimulus based on the rate of activation of an electrode. Commonly, the assigned pitch increases with the rate of stimulation up to about 300 Hz, with no further increases for higher rates of stimulation.

The subjective pitch through an electrode also depends on the position of the electrode in the cochlea, with more basal electrodes giving higher pitches and more apical electrodes giving lower pitches. More apical insertion of electrodes also produces lower perceived pitches (e.g. Hamzavi and Arnoldner, 2006). However, the change with place of stimulation is more commonly described as a change in timbre rather than of pitch itself.

Most patients can accurately rank electrodes in the cochlea according to place of stimulation. Commonly, the change in sensation occurs progressively and relatively smoothly with electrode position along the array, although discontinuities and even reversals are sometimes found. Patients can generally distinguish between the sensations produced by changes in the rate of stimulation and those produced by changes in the place of stimulation, the sensations of which are perceived independently and in a non-interacting way (Tong et al., 1983).

Although available devices contain up to 22 electrodes (i.e. channels), in practice between 8 and 16 electrodes are generally used. The large number of channels potentially available, however, means that the configuration can be optimally selected for each patient, with any high-threshold electrodes, or electrodes that evoke unpleasant effects (e.g. very high pitch; or stimulation of the facial nerve), not being used. The usefulness of an electrode may be affected by, for instance, exactly how the electrode lies within the cochlear duct (e.g. either too near nor too far from the modiolus), survival of the nerve in the region being stimulated and local tissue reaction or bone growth around the electrode. Mapping the effects produced by the different electrodes, including matching the stimulus to the threshold and dynamic range of each electrode, is an essential preliminary step in programming the prosthesis for each patient, and one which has to be repeated regularly during the life of the implant.

10.4.3.3 Perception of complex stimuli

Current devices use variants of a common method of conveying speech. The acoustic stimulus is filtered through multiple bandpass filters (up to 20), with the overall frequency range adjustable for each patient but typically covering the range from 200 Hz to 8 kHz. After filtering, the envelope of the acoustic waveform is calculated for each channel. Those channels with the highest amplitudes are selected, with six channels commonly being chosen. The electrodes are stimulated with brief biphasic current pulses as illustrated in Fig. 10.9, with the amplitude of the pulses presented to any one electrode depending on the amplitude of the acoustic stimulus in the corresponding channel. In some implementations the stimulation is adaptive, with the number of channels selected varying with the number of clear spectral peaks in the stimulus, and with the mapping of the filter bank to the electrode array being dynamically altered to optimize the discriminability of the peaks. Because the amplitude in each channel is calculated at a high rate, and the biphasic pulses are presented at a high rate, the overall stimulation in each channel can follow the rapid temporal fluctuations in the stimulus waveform, while the spatial pattern represents the short-term spectrum of the stimulus.

While the initial sensations through an implant can be perceived as highly unnatural and poor at conveying speech sounds, with practice many patients achieve good speech recognition in quiet with free running speech. Under these circumstances, 80–90% of sentences are recognized correctly, as shown in a summary of published clinical trials (Zeng, 2004). However, in noise, perception drops more rapidly than with normal-hearing subjects, particularly for stimuli containing rapidly changing spectral patterns (Munson and Nelson, 2005).

In cases of partial loss of hearing, acoustic hearing aids are particularly poor at compensating for the losses at high frequencies. Therefore, it can be worth implanting patients with residual low-frequency hearing, a cochlear implant being used to deliver some of the high-frequency information, while an acoustic hearing aid is used to deliver the low-frequency stimuli (e.g. Turner, 2006).

One critical issue is whether stimulation enhances the functional abilities of the auditory nervous system. Animal studies are in conflict as to whether stimulation encourages survival of the remaining auditory nerve fibres, some authors having reported only small effects and others none; the effect therefore seems minor at best (reviewed by Miller, 2001). A further and very critical issue is whether stimulation is necessary for the normal initial development of the central auditory nervous system and whether there is an early critical period for adjusting to stimuli. For these reasons, there is a move towards the early implantation of deaf children. Results are variable; some report that children who are implanted earlier acquire language at a greater rate, while others report that the advantages stem from the greater number of years of use of the implant, with no separate acceleration of learning in most cases (e.g. Cheng *et al.*, 1999; Geers, 2004). There is also evidence that early implantation assists in cognitive functioning, including enhancing visual attention and increasing the speed of verbal articulation which leads to enhanced performance on a range of other tasks (reviewed by Pisoni and Cleary, 2004; see also Horn *et al.*, 2005).

10.5 CELLULAR REPLACEMENT, PROTECTION AND GENE THERAPY IN THE INNER EAR

10.5.1 Introduction

As pointed out above, if hair cells are destroyed in human beings and other mammals they are not replaced. Therefore, it was a surprise to find that in birds, hair cells regenerate after being destroyed by noise or by ototoxic drugs, leading to functional restoration of hearing (Cotanche, 1987; Cruz *et al.*, 1987). This opened the possibility of inducing hair cell regeneration in human beings, prompting the question 'If it works in birds, why not in man?' (Girod and Rubel, 1991).

The aim of restoring functional hearing in human beings has been one of the drivers of a large research effort aimed at discovering the basic developmental programmes that lead to the generation of hair cells and at discovering the genes that control them (Box 10.4; see review by Kelley, 2006).

Box 10.4 · Cell fates in the inner ear

In most cases, many of the genes that control the developmental decisions are known: the reader is referred to the original source for details (Kelley, 2006).

A pointed arrow, Fig. 10.10, indicates that one cell type can develop into another cell type. A flat-ended arrow, Fig. 10.10, indicates that one cell type can inhibit the formation of the other cell type.

Modified and simplified from Kelley (2006), Fig. 5.

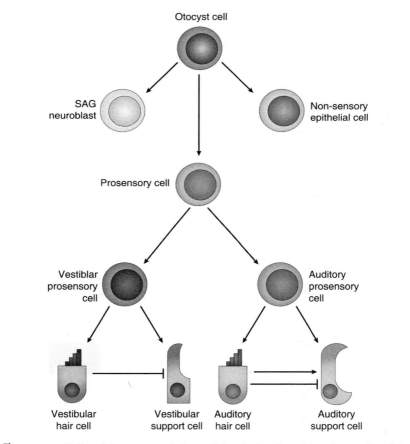

Fig. 10.10 Cells of the otocyst (primordial ear) develop either into cells of the statoacoustic ganglion, prosensory cells or non-sensory cells. Adapted from Kelley (2006), Fig. 5, Copyright (2006), with permission from Macmillan Publishers Ltd, Nature Neuroscience.

The bird cochlea is composed of relatively unspecialized hair cells situated in a simple columnar epithelium. The hair cells do not show the extreme specializations of, for instance, the outer hair cells, nor do the supporting cells show the extreme specialization of the pillar cells or Deiters' cells. It is possible that this unspecialized organization has allowed new hair cells to be produced from supporting cells after damage. Mammalian vestibular organs also have relatively unspecialized sensory epithelia, and adult vestibular epithelia can produce new hair cells after damage, albeit at a low rate (Forge *et al.*, 1993; Oesterle *et al.*, 2003). However, it should be pointed out that mammalian cochlear inner hair cells also appear relatively unspecialized, and they do not regenerate after damage.

10.5.2 Production of new hair cells from supporting cells by mitosis in the mammalian cochlea

In bird cochleae, the regenerated hair cells develop as a result of supporting cells dividing or transdifferentiating (i.e. transforming without cell division) after cochlear damage (Girod *et al.*, 1989; reviewed by Stone and Cotanche, 2007). The hair cells become innervated and are functional (e.g. Wang and Raphael, 1996; Woolley *et al.*, 2001). Can mammalian cochlear supporting cells also be induced to divide and produce new and functional hair cells? The possibility was shown in cultured supporting cells, isolated from the neonatal mouse cochlea. The cells were co-cultured with other cells to promote cellular proliferation and were shown to produce further cells by mitosis (cell division), some of which later developed elementary hair cell-like characteristics (White *et al.*, 2006). However, these results were obtained in vitro using cells from immature cochleae where developmental processes are still continuing, and it is not known whether they will lead to an effective therapy. Supporting cells in the mature guinea pig cochlea have an ability, though a limited one, to proliferate after damage and therefore could possibly provide a source for the new hair cells (Yamasoba and Kondo, 2006). The proliferation of supporting cells is controlled in mammalian cochleae by a cell cycle inhibitor known as $p27^{Kip1}$, and knockout of the $p27^{Kip1}$ gene in mice allows the proliferation of excess supporting cells, with the consequential production of excess hair cells (Chen and Segil, 1999; Lowenheim *et al.*, 1999). However, these animals have severely deformed organs of Corti and severe hearing loss (e.g. Kanzaki *et al.*, 2006a). Nevertheless, the results do suggest that at some time in the future it might be possible to trigger the development of further supporting cells in the organ of Corti and that they could be used as a source for new hair cells.

10.5.3 Production of new hair cells by transdifferentiation of supporting cells

The possibility that mammalian supporting could transdifferentiate directly into hair cells without an intervening mitosis was shown in the vestibular sensory epithelium by Li and Forge (1997). One key gene, *Math-1*, has since been shown to be necessary for the development of hair cells from their precursors (Bermingham *et al.*, 1999). *Math-1* (alternatively called *Atoh 1*) codes for a gene transcription factor. If the *Math-1* gene is introduced into the deafened mammalian cochlea by inoculating the ear with a virus engineered to contain *Math-1*, some supporting cells in the organ of Corti transdifferentiate into hair cells, generating both inner and outer hair cells (Izumikawa *et al.*, 2005). Figure 10.11A shows a scanning electron micrograph of a small region of the organ of Corti of a deafened and inoculated guinea pig, compared with the contralateral cochlea which was deafened but not inoculated (Fig. 10.11B). Figure 10.11C shows that thresholds for auditory brain response, a measure of auditory sensitivity, were lowered in the inoculated

A: SEM Inoculated ear   B: SEM Uninoculated contralateral ear

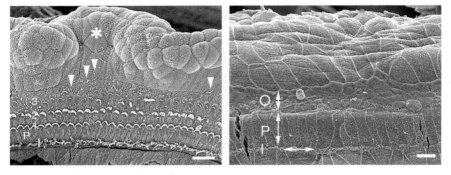

Fig. 10.11   Transdifferentiation of hair cells in the guinea pig organ of Corti following inoculation with *Math-1*. Guinea pigs were first given a combination of kanamycin and ethacrynic acid, which destroyed all inner and outer hair cells in the lower three turns of the cochlea of both ears. Part B shows a scanning electron micrograph of a small region of the organ of Corti of such an ear. All hair cells are lost. One ear in each animal was inoculated with a virus which was engineered to contain the *Math-1* gene. Hair cells reappeared in the inoculated ears (A), but not in the contralateral untreated ears (B). Auditory brainstem responses (ABRs) were lowered in threshold in the inoculated ears (C), but not in the contralateral untreated ears (D). Ears with a greater density of inner hair cells/mm (numbers on curves in part C) had lower ABR thresholds. (A) Inoculated ear, second turn of cochlea, showing transdifferentiated hair cells. 1, 2, 3: 1st, 2nd and 3rd rows of transdifferentiated outer hair cells. I: transdifferentiated inner hair cells. P: pillar cells. Asterisk: site of inoculation. Arrowheads: bundles of stereocilia on ectopic transdifferentiated hair cells, situated outside the normal positions. Scale bar: 25 μm. (B) Untreated ear contralateral to that in part A in the same animal, showing loss of all hair cells. I: inner hair cell area, O: outer hair cell area, P: pillar cells. Scale bar: 10 μm. (C) and (D) Thresholds of ABRs in the treated (C) and untreated (D) ears of the same animals (animals identified by symbol). It is likely that ABR responses due to stimulation of the untreated ears were due to crossed stimulation of the treated ear. The guinea pig with open circle symbols had no detectable responses in response to stimuli applied to the untreated ear. Reprinted from Izumikawa *et al.* (2005), Figs 2A, 2D and 5C, Copyright (2005), with permission from Macmillan Publishers Ltd. Nature Medicine.

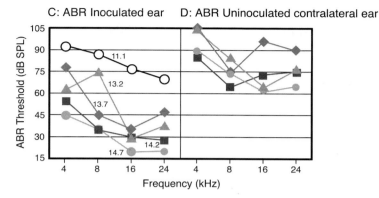

Fig. 10.11 Continued

cochleae, in some animals to near normal, but were high in the contralateral non-inoculated cochleae.

The transdifferentiated cells had many of the cellular and morphological characteristics of hair cells. For instance, they expressed myosin 7A, which is expressed only in hair cells and in the retina, and had many of the morphological features of hair cells, with similar cellular structures and an organized bundle of stereocilia. They also attracted neural dendrites of the spiral ganglion (Kawamoto et al., 2003). While the new inner hair cells appeared normal morphologically, the new outer hair cells appear incompletely differentiated, and therefore may not be fully functional, that is, may not be able to contribute fully to amplifying the mechanical travelling wave and generating normal sensitivity and frequency selectivity.

Moreover, as a result of the transdifferentiation, the normal structure of the organ of Corti, with its array of phalanges of Deiters' cells bracing the upper surface of the organ, is missing. These results were obtained in mature cochleae, in young adult guinea pigs, and form the first findings of the replacement of functional hair cells in the adult cochlea.

10.5.4 Gene therapy

In the cases of inherited hearing losses, there is a theoretical possibility of using gene therapy to prevent the loss in the first place, or of restoring function after the loss has occurred. Gene therapy could consist either of replacing a functional gene, or interfering with the abnormal function of a damaged gene (reviewed by Maiorana and Staecker, 2005). As an example, human DFNB3 is a defect in the gene coding for myosin 15a, with a mouse correlate in the mouse mutant known as *shaker 2*. In a pioneering study, the hearing defect in a *shaker 2* mouse was corrected by making a transgenic mouse that incorporated a normal copy of the myosin 15a gene into its genome. *Shaker 2* mice normally have high auditory thresholds and show circling behaviour, while their hair cells degenerate.

In contrast, the transgenic rescued mice had normal thresholds, normal behaviour and normal cochlear morphology (Probst *et al.*, 1998; Kanzaki *et al.*, 2006b).

10.5.5 Stem cell therapy

Stem cells are cells that have the capacity to self-renew and differentiate into a variety of types of cell. Pluripotent stem cells can be isolated from the cells of the inner cell mass of the blastocyst (precursor of the embryo) to generate a wide range of cell types. Supporting cells from the inner ear can also act as stem cells with more restricted abilities in that they can renew and produce cells that express some of the biochemical markers of hair cells and other types of cells from the inner ear (e.g. Oshima *et al.*, 2007).

Mouse embryonic stem cells can be induced to become hair cell progenitors by treating with a succession of specific growth factors in culture. When implanted into embryonic chicken inner ears, the cells can integrate into the sensory epithelium and develop into hair cells (Li *et al.*, 2003). Neural stem cells, that is, cells that are obtained from mouse embryonic brains and that are already partially committed in their developmental programme, can also integrate into the different epithelia of the inner ear when injected into the mouse cochlea. In most of these cases, the cells become glial or neural cells; however, some cells were found to migrate to the vestibular sensory epithelia and integrate into it, to develop the appearance of hair cells (Tateya *et al.*, 2003). In both of these cases, the cells incorporated into relatively undifferentiated sensory epithelia (see above, Section 10.5.1). Whether incorporation is possible with the more highly specialized organ of Corti is still to be determined.

Stem cells also have the potential for repairing the stria vascularis and the spiral ganglion, also sites of damage in cochlear hearing loss. Stem cells could also be engineered to provide growth factors to support the cells of the spiral ganglion, not only reducing the loss with for instance ageing, but to provide a trophic support for the nerve after implantation of the cochlear prosthesis (Gillespie and Shepherd, 2005).

10.5.6 Cell protection

Although replacing hair cells after they have been lost is a major focus of current effort, protecting hair cells from damage in the first place is a more conservative goal and for that reason may be more achievable. A number of different approaches are under investigation, including chemically protecting the cells from free radicals, identifying and enhancing the cells' own defensive mechanisms, and inhibiting cell death once the cell is damaged.

Free radicals (e.g. reactive oxygen species) are highly damaging to cells. It may therefore be possible to reduce the loss of hair cells by protecting the cells from their effects. Such an effect has been shown conclusively for drug-induced hearing loss in animals, and for aminoglycoside antibiotics in human beings, where aspirin (which is metabolised to an antioxidant) was co-administered with aminoglycoside antibiotics, with a resulting complete protection from ototoxic damage (Sha *et al.*,

2006). Many agents are able to act as antioxidants, and we have the possibility of reducing cell damage in the inner ear, either by applying them directly to the inner ear or applying them systemically (e.g. via the blood stream), so reducing the effects of aminoglycosides, acoustic trauma and possibly ageing (e.g. Lynch and Kil, 2005; see also Forge and Van De Water, 2007 for review).

One enigmatic observation has been that following repeated bouts of acoustic stimulation, the cochlea seems to become more resistant to acoustic damage. The basis for the phenomenon, known as sound conditioning or toughening, is not clear. Enhanced antioxidant defences may be part of the explanation, because following sound conditioning, not only do antioxidant enzymes increase in the inner ear but the ear develops an increased resistance to oxidative attack by externally applied chemical agents (Harris et al., 2006). The phenomenon may have mechanisms in common with the effects of heat stress, since hyperthermia can also make the ear more resistant to acoustic trauma. Heat induces the production of heat shock proteins, which can have a variety of effects in the cochlea, including acting as antioxidants, protecting proteins from damage, and suppressing apoptotic pathways (reviewed by Altschuler et al., 2002).

Damage to the hair cells may initiate a sequence of events leading either to necrosis or to programmed cell death (apoptosis). This is presumably appropriate if the cells can be replaced by mitosis, and therefore may be a general mechanism favoured by evolution for that reason. However, if the cell cannot be replaced, it may not be advantageous, and under these circumstances, it may be more favourable to inhibit apoptosis. In cultures of mammalian or bird vestibular epithelia, inhibition of cell death pathways can lead to survival of hair cells after an aminoglycoside insult that otherwise would have been lethal to the cells (Forge and Li, 2000; Cheng et al., 2005). Similarly, cells of the spiral ganglion can survive in culture condition under which they would otherwise die, if pro-survival members of the pathways controlling apoptosis are overexpressed in the cells (Hansen et al., 2007). The results suggest that the extent of apoptosis after insults to the inner ear may not always be at a level that is optimal for the organism and that the survival of functional hair cells and cells of the spiral ganglion can be enhanced by reducing the extent of apoptosis in the cochlea.

10.6 SUMMARY

1. Hearing loss can arise in the conductive apparatus before the oval window, when it is known as conductive loss. Alternatively, it may arise in the cochlea or more centrally, when it is known as sensorineural hearing loss. If it arises in the cochlea, it is known as sensorineural hearing loss of cochlear origin.
2. Sensorineural hearing loss of cochlear origin can be caused by ototoxic drugs. Aminoglycoside antibiotics are ototoxic and have been extensively investigated, although we are still unclear as to their precise mechanisms of ototoxicity. Aminoglycosides damage hair cells, and particularly outer hair cells,

in the high-frequency parts of the cochlea. They may cause their damage by oxidative mechanisms, and antioxidants can provide some protection.

3. Other ototoxic agents include Cisplatin (an anticancer drug), some loop diuretics (bumetanide, furosemide and ethacrynic acid), aspirin (reversibly) and some organic solvents (e.g. styrene and toluene).

4. With acoustic overstimulation, for milder degrees of damage, there is minor disruption of the stereocilia. These degrees of damage are probably reversible. Greater degrees of damage cause loss of the hair cells.

5. Hearing losses may also have genetic causes. The commonest inherited hearing loss, accounting for some 35% of all congenital hearing losses (depending on the population), is the type known as DFNB1. DFNB1 is caused by a mutation in the gene coding for the gap junction protein connexin-26. Patients with this mutation have problems cycling K^+ from the cochlear scalae through the cochlear walls back to the stria vascularis. This and many other inherited hearing losses have been invaluable for revealing basic mechanisms of the inner ear.

6. Mutations in the mitochondrial genome may also give rise to hearing loss. These syndromes are maternally inherited, commonly affect multiple organ systems, and tend to increase with severity over time.

7. Ageing causes sensorineural hearing loss (presbyacusis), which can have both cochlear and central components. In the cochlea, vulnerable sites are the hair cells, the nerve and the stria vascularis.

8. Damage to the outer hair cells causes a loss of the active amplification of the mechanical travelling wave in the cochlear duct. This leads to a reduction in the magnitude of the travelling wave and a broadening of the peak of the wave. The changes lead to a loss in the sensitivity of auditory nerve fibres, and a broadening of their tuning curves, that is, to a loss of frequency resolution. Damage to the inner hair cells leads to a loss of sensitivity of the auditory nerve fibres, without changes in frequency resolution.

9. The psychophysical results fit in with the physiological results. In sensorineural loss of cochlear origin, a loss of frequency resolution is often seen in addition to the loss in sensitivity. The loss in frequency resolution can be seen in widened psychophysical tuning curves and in widened psychophysical filters (critical bands). These factors lead to a particular difficulty in understanding broadband complex sounds, such as speech, and particularly against noisy backgrounds.

10. Some forms of tinnitus, that is, those arise in the cochlea from the active mechanical amplification of the travelling wave, may give rise to objectively measurable sound emissions in the ear canal. However, this is unlikely to explain the clinically most important forms of tinnitus. Tinnitus is commonly associated with some degree of hearing loss. This suggests that it arises from a hypersensitivity of the central auditory nervous system when it is deprived of its normal input. It appears that neural activity increases in the extralemniscal auditory pathway (which starts in the dorsal cochlear nucleus), that is, the less specific auditory nuclei which are situated alongside the specific, or lemniscal, auditory nuclei. The extralemniscal nuclei often generate arousing or alerting responses to auditory stimuli, which may account for the intrusive nature

of tinnitus. The tinnitus may arise from a reduction in inhibition by the neurotransmitter GABA in the extralemniscal nuclei, and a drug vigabatrin that increases GABA levels has been reported to reverse tinnitus in experimental animals. In the absence of a current effective drug treatment in human beings, the behavioural method known as 'tinnitus retraining therapy' has proved effective in many patients.

11. With profound sensorineural hearing loss of cochlear origin, hearing can often be restored by a cochlear prosthesis. Current prostheses consist of multiple electrodes inserted deep into the cochlear duct, where they can stimulate what cells remain of the auditory nerve. Stimuli are pre-processed to pick out the major spectral components of the stimuli, and electrodes at the appropriate positions in the cochlea (depending on the tonotopicity of the cochlea) are stimulated electrically. The amplitude of stimulation depends on the amplitude of the relevant spectral component at each moment, so that the final pattern of stimulation is able to mirror both the place-frequency and temporal aspects of cochlear function. After practice, 80–90% of open-set sentences are understood correctly.

12. Attempts are being made to replace damaged cells in the inner ear, including the hair cells, cells of the spiral ganglion (auditory nerve) and the stria vascularis. These include (i) stimulating the division of the supporting cells, to produce new hair cells; (ii) inoculating the cochlea with a virus engineered to contain a gene *math-1*, which encourages the supporting cells to transdifferentiate (i.e. transform without undergoing cell division) into hair cells and (iii) the injection of stem cells. The transdifferentiation of supporting cells induced by *math-1* has been able to partially restore some hearing in adult animals even after complete loss of all hair cells.

13. Gene therapy may be possible, where the function of a damaged gene is replaced by an introduced normal copy of the gene. Protection of hair cells may also be possible by (i) inhibiting apoptotic pathways, (ii) use of antioxidant therapy and (iii) manipulations which increase the ear's own biochemical protective mechanisms, for example, those arising in the phenomenon known as 'sound conditioning' or 'toughening', and those which increase the levels of heat shock proteins to generate a variety of protective effects.

10.7 FURTHER READING

Aminoglycoside ototoxicity has been reviewed by Forge and Schacht (2000). Cisplatin ototoxicity has been reviewed by Rybak *et al.* (2007). Noise-induced hearing loss has been reviewed by Henderson *et al.* (2006).

The genetics of deafness has been reviewed by Finsterer and Fellinger (2005), Schrijver and Gardner (2006), Petersen and Willems (2006) and by Petit (2006). Ohlemiller (2006) discusses the contributions of mouse models to understanding hearing loss. Mitochondrial involvement has been reviewed by Finsterer and

Fellinger (2005), Fischel-Ghodsian *et al.* (2004), Pickles (2004) and Hutchin and Cortopassi (2000).

Tinnitus has been reviewed in a special issue of Acta Otolaryngologica, Supplement 556 (vol. 126, 2006), pp. 1–105 and by Eggermont (2005). Tinnitus retraining therapy has been reviewed by Jastreboff and Jastreboff (2006).

Fundamental psychophysical changes in hearing loss have been reviewed by Moore (2005).

For cochlear prostheses, several chapters of 'Cochlear Implants: Auditory Prostheses and Electric Hearing' (eds F.G. Zeng, A.N. Popper and R.R Fay; Springer Handbook of Auditory Research, vol 20, 2004) are valuable, as well as a review by Rubinstein (2004). Otolaryngological journals have regular special issues on recent advances in cochlear implantation which should be sought out, for example, 'Cochlear and Brainstem Implants' (Advances in Otorhinolaryngology, vol. 64, pp. 1–258, 2006, ed. A.R. Moller).

Hair cell development has been reviewed by Kelley (2006) and Kros (2007), and in many chapters of 'Development of the Ear' (edited by M. W. Kelley, D. K. Wu, A. N. Popper, R. R. Fay; Springer Handbook of Auditory Research, vol. 26, 2005).

Stem cells and hair cell regeneration and transdifferentiation have also been reviewed in 'Regeneration and Repair' (eds R. J. Salvi, A. N. Popper and R. R. Fay; Springer Handbook of Auditory Research, vol 33, 2008), and also by Parker and Cotanche (2004), Matsui and Ryals (2005) and Batts and Raphael (2007). Repair of the nerve has been further reviewed by Gillespie and Shepherd (2005) and by Roehm and Hansen (2005). Hair cell death and protection have been reviewed by Cheng *et al.* (2005) and Forge and Van De Water (2007).

References

Abeles, M., Goldstein, M.H., Jr. 1972. Responses of single units in the primary auditory cortex of the cat to tones and to tone pairs. Brain Res 42, 337–352.

Abrashkin, K.A., Izumikawa, M., Miyazawa, T., Wang, C.H., Crumling, M.A., Swiderski, D.L., Beyer, L.A., Gong, T.W., Raphael, Y. 2006. The fate of outer hair cells after acoustic or ototoxic insults. Hear Res 218, 20–29.

Adams, J.C. 1979. Ascending projections to the inferior colliculus. J Comp Neurol 183, 519–538.

Adams, J.C., Mugnaini, E. 1984. Dorsal nucleus of the lateral lemniscus: a nucleus of GABAergic projection neurons. Brain Res Bull 13, 585–590.

Ahveninen, J., Jaaskelainen, I.P., Raij, T., Bonmassar, G., Devore, S., Hamalainen, M., Levanen, S., Lin, F.H., Sams, M., Shinn-Cunningham, B.G., Witzel, T., Belliveau, J.W. 2006. Task-modulated "what" and "where" pathways in human auditory cortex. Proc Natl Acad Sci USA 103, 14608–14613.

Aibara, R., Welsh, J.T., Puria, S., Goode, R.L. 2001. Human middle-ear sound transfer function and cochlear input impedance. Hear Res 152, 100–109.

Aitkin, L.M. 1973. Medial geniculate body of the cat: responses to tonal stimuli of neurons in medial division. J Neurophysiol 36, 275–283.

Aitkin, L.M., Prain, S.M. 1974. Medial geniculate body: unit responses in the awake cat. J Neurophysiol 37, 512–521.

Aitkin, L.M., Webster, W.R. 1972. Medial geniculate body of the cat: organization and responses to tonal stimuli of neurons in ventral division. J Neurophysiol 35, 365–380.

Aitkin, L.M., Webster, W.R., Veale, J.L., Crosby, D.C. 1975. Inferior colliculus. I. Comparison of response properties of neurons in central, pericentral, and external nuclei of adult cat. J Neurophysiol 38, 1196–1207.

Aitkin, L.M., Dickhaus, H., Schult, W., Zimmermann, M. 1978. External nucleus of inferior colliculus: auditory and spinal somatosensory afferents and their interactions. J Neurophysiol 41, 837–847.

Alibardi, L. 2002. Putative inhibitory collicular boutons contact large neurons and their dendrites in the dorsal cochlear nucleus of the rat. J Submicrosc Cytol Pathol 34, 433–446.

Alkhatib, A., Biebel, U.W., Smolders, J.W. 2006. Inhibitory and excitatory response areas of neurons in the central nucleus of the inferior colliculus in unanesthetized chinchillas. Exp Brain Res 174, 124–143.

Altschuler, R.A., Fairfield, D., Cho, Y., Leonova, E., Benjamin, I.J., Miller, J.M., Lomax, M.I. 2002. Stress pathways in the rat cochlea and potential for protection from acquired deafness. Audiol Neurootol 7, 152–156.

Andrews, J.C. 2004. Intralabyrinthine fluid dynamics: Meniere disease. Curr Opin Otolaryngol Head Neck Surg 12, 408–412.

Anniko, M., Wroblewski, R. 1986. Ionic environment of cochlear hair cells. Hear Res 22, 279–293.

Arnott, R.H., Wallace, M.N., Shackleton, T.M., Palmer, A.R. 2004a. Onset neurones in the anteroventral cochlear nucleus project to the dorsal cochlear nucleus. J Assoc Res Otolaryngol 5, 153–170.

Arnott, S.R., Binns, M.A., Grady, C.L., Alain, C. 2004b. Assessing the auditory dual-pathway model in humans. Neuroimage 22, 401–408.

Arthur, R.M., Pfeiffer, R.R., Suga, N. 1971. Properties of 'two-tone inhibition' in primary auditory neurones. J Physiol 212, 593–609.

Assad, J.A., Shepherd, G.M., Corey, D.P. 1991. Tip-link integrity and mechanical transduction in vertebrate hair cells. Neuron 7, 985–994.

Avan, P., Bonfils, P. 1992. Analysis of possible interactions of an attentional task with cochlear micromechanics. Hear Res 57, 269–275.

Bacon, S.P., Moore, B.C. 1986. Temporal effects in masking and their influence on psychophysical tuning curves. J Acoust Soc Am 80, 1638–1645.

Banks, W.F., Saunders, J.C., Lowry, L.D. 1979. Olivocochlear bundle activity recorded in awake cats. Otolaryngol Head Neck Surg 87, 463–471.

Barrett, D.J., Hall, D.A. 2006. Response preferences for "what" and "where" in human non-primary auditory cortex. Neuroimage 32, 968–977.

Batts, S.A., Raphael, Y. 2007. Transdifferentiation and its applicability for inner ear therapy. Hear Res 227, 41–47.

Bauer, J.W. 1978. Tuning curves and masking functions of auditory-nerve fibers in cat. Sens Processes 2, 156–172.

Beckius, G.E., Batra, R., Oliver, D.L. 1999. Axons from anteroventral cochlear nucleus that terminate in medial superior olive of cat: observations related to delay lines. J Neurosci 19, 3146–3161.

Behne, N., Wendt, B., Scheich, H., Brechmann, A. 2006. Contralateral white noise selectively changes left human auditory cortex activity in a lexical decision task. J Neurophysiol 95, 2630–2637.

Békésy, G. von. 1947. The variation in phase along the basilar membrane with sinusoidal vibrations. J Acoust Soc Am 19, 452–460.

Békésy, G. von. 1949. On the resonance curve and the decay period at various points on the cochlear partition. J Acoust Soc Am 21, 245–254.

Békésy, G. von. 1953. Description of some mechanical properties of the organ of Corti. J Acoust Soc Am 25, 770–785.

Békésy, G. von. 1960. Experiments in Hearing (Wever, E.G., Ed.). McGraw-Hill, New York. Reissued 1989, Acoustical Society of America.

van Bergeijk, W.A. 1962. Variation on a theme of von Békésy: a model of binaural interaction. J Acoust Soc Am 34, 1431–1437.

Bermingham, N.A., Hassan, B.A., Price, S.D., Vollrath, M.A., Ben-Arie, N., Eatock, R.A., Bellen, H.J., Lysakowski, A., Zoghbi, H.Y. 1999. Math1: an essential gene for the generation of inner ear hair cells. Science 284, 1837–1841.

Beurg, M., Evans, M.G., Hackney, C.M., Fettiplace, R. 2006. A large-conductance calcium-selective mechanotransducer channel in mammalian cochlear hair cells. J Neurosci 26, 10992–11000.

Biebel, U.W., Langner, G. 2002. Evidence for interactions across frequency channels in the inferior colliculus of awake chinchilla. Hear Res 169, 151–168.

Billig, I., Yeager, M.S., Blikas, A., Raz, Y. 2007. Neurons in the cochlear nuclei controlling the tensor tympani muscle in the rat: A study using pseudorabies virus. Brain Res 1154, 124–136.

Binns, K.E., Grant, S., Withington, D.J., Keating, M.J. 1992. A topographic representation of auditory space in the external nucleus of the inferior colliculus of the guinea-pig. Brain Res 589, 231–242.

Birt, D., Nienhuis, R., Olds, M. 1979. Separation of associative from non-associative short latency changes in medial geniculate and inferior colliculus during differential conditioning and reversal in rats. Brain Res 167, 129–138.

Blackburn, C.C., Sachs, M.B. 1990. The representations of the steady-state vowel sound /ɛ/ in the discharge patterns of cat anteroventral cochlear nucleus neurons. J Neurophysiol 63, 1191–1212.

Blauert, J. 1997. Spatial Hearing: The Psychophysics of Human Sound Localization. MIT Press, Cambridge.

Boatman, D.F. 2006. Cortical auditory systems: speech and other complex sounds. Epilepsy Behav 8, 494–503.

Boeda, B., El-Amraoui, A., Bahloul, A., Goodyear, R., Daviet, L., Blanchard, S., Perfettini, I., Fath, K.R., Shorte, S., Reiners, J., Houdusse, A., Legrain, P., Wolfrum, U., Richardson, G., Petit, C. 2002. Myosin VIIa, harmonin and cadherin 23, three Usher I gene products that cooperate to shape the sensory hair cell bundle. Embo J 21, 6689–6699.

de Boer, E. 1996. Mechanics of the cochlea: modeling efforts. In: Dallos, P., Popper, A.N., Fay, R.R. (Eds), The Cochlea, Springer Handbook of Auditory Research, Vol. 8. Springer, New York. pp. 258–317.

de Boer, E., de Jongh, H.R. 1978. On cochlear encoding: potentialities and limitations of the reverse-correlation technique. J Acoust Soc Am 63, 115–135.

de Boer, E., Nuttall, A.L. 1999. The "inverse problem" solved for a three-dimensional model of the cochlea. III. Brushing-up the solution method. J Acoust Soc Am 105, 3410–3420.

de Boer, E., Nuttall, A.L. 2002. Properties of amplifying elements in the cochlea. In: Gummer, A.W., Dalhoff, E., Nowotny, M., Scherer, M.P. (Eds), Biophysics of the Cochlea: From Molecules to Models. World Scientific, Singapore. pp. 331–342.

Boudreau, J.C., Tsuchitani, C. 1968. Binaural interaction in the cat superior olive S segment. J Neurophysiol 31, 442–454.

Brand, A., Behrend, O., Marquardt, T., McAlpine, D., Grothe, B. 2002. Precise inhibition is essential for microsecond interaural time difference coding. Nature 417, 543–547.

Brodmann, K. 1909. Vergleichende Localisationslehre der Grosshirnrinde, Barth, Leipzig (Eng. Tr. as Localisation in the Cerebral Cortex; by Garey, L.J., 1994, Smith-Gordon, London).

Brown, M.C. 1987. Morphology of labeled afferent fibers in the guinea pig cochlea. J Comp Neurol 260, 591–604.

Brown, M.C. 1989. Morphology and response properties of single olivocochlear fibers in the guinea pig. Hear Res 40, 93–109.

Brown, M.C., Nuttall, A.L. 1984. Efferent control of cochlear inner hair cell responses in the guinea-pig. J Physiol 354, 625–646.

Brown, A.M., Pye, J.D. 1975. Auditory sensitivity at high frequencies in mammals. Adv Comp Physiol Biochem 6, 1–73.

Brown, M.C., Nuttall, A.L., Masta, R.I. 1983. Intracellular recordings from cochlear inner hair cells: effects of stimulation of the crossed olivocochlear efferents. Science 222, 69–72.

Brown, M., Webster, W.R., Martin, R.L. 1997. The three-dimensional frequency organization of the inferior colliculus of the cat: a 2-deoxyglucose study. Hear Res 104, 57–72.

Brownell, W.E., Bader, C.R., Bertrand, D., de Ribaupierre, Y. 1985. Evoked mechanical responses of isolated cochlear outer hair cells. Science 227, 194–196.

Brozoski, T.J., Spires, T.J., Bauer, C.A. 2007. Vigabatrin, a GABA transaminase inhibitor, reversibly eliminates tinnitus in an animal model. J Assoc Res Otolaryngol 8, 105–118.

Brugge, J.F., Reale, R.A., Hind, J.E., Chan, J.C., Musicant, A.D., Poon, P.W. 1994. Simulation of free-field sound sources and its application to studies of cortical mechanisms of sound localization in the cat. Hear Res 73, 67–84.

Brugge, J.F., Reale, R.A., Hind, J.E. 1996. The structure of spatial receptive fields of neurons in primary auditory cortex of the cat. J Neurosci 16, 4420–4437.

Burnett, L.R., Stein, B.E., Chaponis, D., Wallace, M.T. 2004. Superior colliculus lesions preferentially disrupt multisensory orientation. Neuroscience 124, 535–547.

Buunen, T.J., Vlaming, M.S. 1981. Laser–Doppler velocity meter applied to tympanic membrane vibrations in cat. J Acoust Soc Am 69, 744–750.

Caird, D., Klinke, R. 1983. Processing of binaural stimuli by cat superior olivary complex neurons. Exp Brain Res 52, 385–399.

Cajal, S.R. 1909. Histologie du Système Nerveux de l'Homme et des Vertébres. Maloine, Paris, Reissued (Eng. Tr. by Swanson, N. and Swanson, L., 1995, Oxford University Press, New York).

Calford, M.B. 1983. The parcellation of the medial geniculate body of the cat defined by the auditory response properties of single units. J Neurosci 3, 2350–2364.

Calford, M.B., Aitkin, L.M. 1983. Ascending projections to the medial geniculate body of the cat: evidence for multiple, parallel auditory pathways through thalamus. J Neurosci 3, 2365–2380.

Calford, M.B., Webster, W.R., Semple, M.M. 1983. Measurement of frequency selectivity of single neurons in the central auditory pathway. Hear Res 11, 395–401.

Campbell, R.A., Doubell, T.P., Nodal, F.R., Schnupp, J.W., King, A.J. 2006. Interaural timing cues do not contribute to the map of space in the ferret superior colliculus: a virtual acoustic space study. J Neurophysiol 95, 242–254.

Cant, N.B., Benson, C.G. 2003. Parallel auditory pathways: projection patterns of the different neuronal populations in the dorsal and ventral cochlear nuclei. Brain Res Bull 60, 457–474.

Cant, N.B., Morest, D.K. 1978. Axons from non-cochlear sources in the anteroventral cochlear nucleus of the cat. A study with the rapid Golgi method. Neuroscience 3, 1003–1029.

Carmel, P.W., Starr, A. 1963. Acoustic and nonacoustic factors modifying middle-ear muscle activity in waking cats. J Neurophysiol 26, 598–616.

Carney, A.E., Nelson, D.A. 1983. An analysis of psychophysical tuning curves in normal and pathological ears. J Acoust Soc Am 73, 268–278.

Caspary, D.M., Havey, D.C., Faingold, C.L. 1983. Effects of acetylcholine on cochlear nucleus neurons. Exp Neurol 82, 491–498.

Caspary, D.M., Backoff, P.M., Finlayson, P.G., Palombi, P.S. 1994. Inhibitory inputs modulate discharge rate within frequency receptive fields of anteroventral cochlear nucleus neurons. J Neurophysiol 72, 2124–2133.

Caspary, D.M., Milbrandt, J.C., Helfert, R.H. 1995. Central auditory aging: GABA changes in the inferior colliculus. Exp Gerontol 30, 349–360.

Caspary, D.M., Palombi, P.S., Hughes, L.F. 2002. GABAergic inputs shape responses to amplitude modulated stimuli in the inferior colliculus. Hear Res 168, 163–173.

Casseday, J.H., Fremouw, T., Covey, E. 2002. The inferior colliculus: a hub for the central nervous system. In: Oertel, D., Fay, R.R., Popper, A.N. (Eds), Integrative Functions in the Mammalian Auditory Pathway, Springer Handbook of Auditory Research, Vol. 15. Springer, New York. pp. 238–318.

Cetas, J.S., Price, R.O., Velenovsky, D.S., Sinex, D.G., McMullen, N.T. 2001. Frequency organization and cellular lamination in the medial geniculate body of the rabbit. Hear Res 155, 113–123.

Cetas, J.S., Price, R.O., Velenovsky, D.S., Crowe, J.J., Sinex, D.G., McMullen, N.T. 2002. Cell types and response properties of neurons in the ventral division of the medial geniculate body of the rabbit. J Comp Neurol 445, 78–96.

Cetas, J.S., Price, R.O., Crowe, J., Velenovsky, D.S., McMullen, N.T. 2003. Dendritic orientation and laminar architecture in the rabbit auditory thalamus. J Comp Neurol 458, 307–317.

Chase, S.M., Young, E.D. 2005. Limited segregation of different types of sound localization information among classes of units in the inferior colliculus. J Neurosci 25, 7575–7585.

Cheatham, M.A., Dallos, P. 1997. Intermodulation components in inner hair cell and organ of Corti responses. J Acoust Soc Am 102, 1038–1048.

Cheatham, M.A., Dallos, P. 1999. Response phase: a view from the inner hair cell. J Acoust Soc Am 105, 799–810.

Cheatham, M.A., Dallos, P. 2000. The dynamic range of inner hair cell and organ of Corti responses. J Acoust Soc Am 107, 1508–1520.

Cheatham, M.A., Dallos, P. 2001. Inner hair cell response patterns: implications for low-frequency hearing. J Acoust Soc Am 110, 2034–2044.

Chen, P., Segil, N. 1999. p27(Kip1) links cell proliferation to morphogenesis in the developing organ of Corti. Development 126, 1581–1590.

Cheng, A.K., Grant, G.D., Niparko, J.K. 1999. Meta-analysis of pediatric cochlear implant literature. Ann Otol Rhinol Laryngol Suppl 177, 124–128.

Cheng, A.G., Cunningham, L.L., Rubel, E.W. 2005. Mechanisms of hair cell death and protection. Curr Opin Otolaryngol Head Neck Surg 13, 343–348.

Cheung, E.L., Corey, D.P. 2006. Ca^{2+} changes the force sensitivity of the hair-cell transduction channel. Biophys J 90, 124–139.

Cheung, S.W., Bedenbaugh, P.H., Nagarajan, S.S., Schreiner, C.E. 2001. Functional organization of squirrel monkey primary auditory cortex: responses to pure tones. J Neurophysiol 85, 1732–1749.

Choudhury, N., Song, G., Chen, F., Matthews, S., Tschinkel, T., Zheng, J., Jacques, S.L., Nuttall, A.L. 2006. Low coherence interferometry of the cochlear partition. Hear Res 220, 1–9.

Christensen, A.P., Corey, D.P. 2007. TRP channels in mechanosensation: direct or indirect activation? Nat Rev Neurosci 8, 510–521.

Clarey, J.C., Irvine, D.R. 1990. The anterior ectosylvian sulcal auditory field in the cat: I. An electrophysiological study of its relationship to surrounding auditory cortical fields. J Comp Neurol 301, 289–303.

Clarey, J.C., Barone, P., Imig, T.J. 1992. Physiology of thalamus and cortex. In: Popper, A.N., Fay, R.R. (Eds), The Mammalian Auditory Pathway: Neurophysiology, Springer Handbook of Auditory Research, Vol. 2. Springer, New York. pp. 232–334.

Clark, J.A., Pickles, J.O. 1996. The effects of moderate and low levels of acoustic overstimulation on stereocilia and their tip links in the guinea pig. Hear Res 99, 119–128.

Code, R.A., Winer, J.A. 1986. Columnar organization and reciprocity of commissural connections in cat primary auditory cortex (AI). Hear Res 23, 205–222.

Cody, A.R., Russell, I.J. 1987. The response of hair cells in the basal turn of the guinea-pig cochlea to tones. J Physiol 383, 551–569.

Cohen, L.T., Saunders, E., Clark, G.M. 2001. Psychophysics of a prototype peri-modiolar cochlear implant electrode array. Hear Res 155, 63–81.

Colburn, H.S., Durlach, N.I. 1978. Models of binaural interaction. In: Carterette, E., Friedman, M. (Eds), Handbook of Perception: Hearing, Vol. 4. Academic Press, New York. pp. 467–518.

Colburn, H.S., Kulikarni, A. 2005. Models of sound localization. In: Popper, A.N., Fay, R.R. (Eds), Sound Source Localization, Springer Handbook of Auditory Research, Vol. 25. Springer, New York. pp. 272–316.

Colburn, H.S., Carney, L.H., Heinz, M.G. 2003. Quantifying the information in auditory-nerve responses for level discrimination. J Assoc Res Otolaryngol 4, 294–311.

Comis, S.D. 1970. Centrifugal inhibitory processes affecting neurones in the cat cochlear nucleus. J Physiol 210, 751–760.

Comis, S.D., Whitfield, I.C. 1968. Influence of centrifugal pathways on unit activity in the cochlear nucleus. J Neurophysiol 31, 62–68.

Comis, S.D., Pickles, J.O., Osborne, M.P. 1985. Osmium tetroxide postfixation in relation to the crosslinkage and spatial organization of stereocilia in the guinea-pig cochlea. J Neurocytol 14, 113–130.

Coomes, D.L., Schofield, B.R. 2004. Separate projections from the inferior colliculus to the cochlear nucleus and thalamus in guinea pigs. Hear Res 191, 67–78.

Cooper, N.P. 1998. Harmonic distortion on the basilar membrane in the basal turn of the guinea-pig cochlea. J Physiol 509, 277–288.

Cooper, N.P., Guinan, J.J., Jr. 2003. Separate mechanical processes underlie fast and slow effects of medial olivocochlear efferent activity. J Physiol 548, 307–312.

Cooper, N.P., Guinan, J.J., Jr. 2006. Efferent-mediated control of basilar membrane motion. J Physiol 576, 49–54.

Cooper, N.P., Rhode, W.S. 1997. Mechanical responses to two-tone distortion products in the apical and basal turns of the mammalian cochlea. J Neurophysiol 78, 261–270.

Corey, D.P. 2006. What is the hair cell transduction channel? J Physiol 576, 23–8.

Corey, D.P., Hudspeth, A.J. 1979a. Ionic basis of the receptor potential in a vertebrate hair cell. Nature 281, 675–677.

Corey, D.P., Hudspeth, A.J. 1979b. Response latency of vertebrate hair cells. Biophys J 26, 499–506.

Corey, D.P., Hudspeth, A.J. 1983. Kinetics of the receptor current in bullfrog saccular hair cells. J Neurosci 3, 962–976.

Corey, D.P., Garcia-Anoveros, J., Holt, J.R., Kwan, K.Y., Lin, S.Y., Vollrath, M.A., Amalfitano, A., Cheung, E.L., Derfler, B.H., Duggan, A., Geleoc, G.S., Gray, P.A., Hoffman, M.P., Rehm, H.L., Tamasauskas, D., Zhang, D.S. 2004. TRPA1 is a candidate for the mechanosensitive transduction channel of vertebrate hair cells. Nature 432, 723–730.

Costalupes, J.A., Young, E.D., Gibson, D.J. 1984. Effects of continuous noise backgrounds on rate response of auditory nerve fibers in cat. J Neurophysiol 51, 1326–1344.

Cotanche, D.A. 1987. Regeneration of hair cell stereociliary bundles in the chick cochlea following severe acoustic trauma. Hear Res 30, 181–195.

Cotanche, D.A., Lee, K.H., Stone, J.S., Picard, D.A. 1994. Hair cell regeneration in the bird cochlea following noise damage or ototoxic drug damage. Anat Embryol (Berl) 189, 1–18.

Counter, S.A., Borg, E. 1993. Acoustic middle ear muscle reflex protection against magnetic coil impulse noise. Acta Otolaryngol 113, 483–488.

Crawford, A.C., Fettiplace, R. 1985. The mechanical properties of ciliary bundles of turtle cochlear hair cells. J Physiol 364, 359–379.

Crawford, A.C., Evans, M.G., Fettiplace, R. 1991. The actions of calcium on the mechano-electrical transducer current of turtle hair cells. J Physiol 434, 369–398.

Crinion, J.T., Lambon-Ralph, M.A., Warburton, E.A., Howard, D., Wise, R.J. 2003. Temporal lobe regions engaged during normal speech comprehension. Brain 126, 1193–1201.

Cruz, R.M., Lambert, P.R., Rubel, E.W. 1987. Light microscopic evidence of hair cell regeneration after gentamicin toxicity in chick cochlea. Arch Otolaryngol Head Neck Surg 113, 1058–1062.

Dallos, P. 1985. Response characteristics of mammalian cochlear hair cells. J Neurosci 5, 1591–1608.

Dallos, P. 1986. Neurobiology of cochlear inner and outer hair cells: intracellular recordings. Hear Res 22, 185–198.

Dallos, P., Evans, B.N. 1995a. High-frequency motility of outer hair cells and the cochlear amplifier. Science 267, 2006–2009.

Dallos, P., Evans, B.N. 1995b. High-frequency outer hair cell motility: corrections and addendum. Science 268, 1420–1421.

Dallos, P., Billone, M.C., Durrant, J.D., Wang, C., Raynor, S. 1972. Cochlear inner and outer hair cells: functional differences. Science 177, 356–358.

Dallos, P., Santos-Sacchi, J., Flock, A. 1982. Intracellular recordings from cochlear outer hair cells. Science 218, 582–584.

Dallos, P., Zheng, J., Cheatham, M.A. 2006. Prestin and the cochlear amplifier. J Physiol 576, 37–42.

D'Angelo, W.R., Sterbing, S.J., Ostapoff, E.M., Kuwada, S. 2005. Role of GABAergic inhibition in the coding of interaural time differences of low-frequency sounds in the inferior colliculus. J Neurophysiol 93, 3390–3400.

Darrow, K.N., Maison, S.F., Liberman, M.C. 2006a. Cochlear efferent feedback balances interaural sensitivity. Nat Neurosci 9, 1474–1476.

Darrow, K.N., Simons, E.J., Dodds, L., Liberman, M.C. 2006b. Dopaminergic innervation of the mouse inner ear: evidence for a separate cytochemical group of cochlear efferent fibers. J Comp Neurol 498, 403–414.

Darrow, K.N., Maison, S.F., Liberman, M.C. 2007. Selective removal of lateral olivo-cochlear efferents increases vulnerability to acute acoustic injury. J Neurophysiol 97, 1775–1785.

Davis, H. 1958. Transmission and transduction in the cochlea. Laryngoscope 68, 359–382.

Davis, K.A., Ramachandran, R., May, B.J. 1999. Single-unit responses in the inferior colliculus of decerebrate cats. II. Sensitivity to interaural level differences. J Neurophysiol 82, 164–175.

Dean, I., Harper, N.S., McAlpine, D. 2005. Neural population coding of sound level adapts to stimulus statistics. Nat Neurosci 8, 1684–1689.

DeBello, W.M., Knudsen, E.I. 2004. Multiple sites of adaptive plasticity in the owl's auditory localization pathway. J Neurosci 24, 6853–6861.

Dehner, L.R., Keniston, L.P., Clemo, H.R., Meredith, M.A. 2004. Cross-modal circuitry between auditory and somatosensory areas of the cat anterior ectosylvian sulcal cortex: a 'new' inhibitory form of multisensory convergence. Cereb Cortex 14, 387–403.

Delano, P.H., Elgueda, D., Hamame, C.M., Robles, L. 2007. Selective attention to visual stimuli reduces cochlear sensitivity in chinchillas. J Neurosci 27, 4146–4153.

Delgutte, B., Kiang, N.Y. 1984a. Speech coding in the auditory nerve: I. Vowel-like sounds. J Acoust Soc Am 75, 866–878.

Delgutte, B., Kiang, N.Y. 1984b. Speech coding in the auditory nerve: III. Voiceless fricative consonants. J Acoust Soc Am 75, 887–896.

Delgutte, B., Hammond, B.M., Cariani, P.A. 1998. Neural coding of the temporal envelope of speech: relation to modulation transfer functions. In: Palmer, A.R., Rees, A., Summerfield, A.Q., Meddis, R. (Eds), Psychophysical and Physiological Advances in Hearing. Whurr, London. pp. 595–602.

Démonet, J.F., Thierry, G., Cardebat, D. 2005. Renewal of the neurophysiology of language: functional neuroimaging. Physiol Rev 85, 49–95.

Denk, W., Holt, J.R., Shepherd, G.M., Corey, D.P. 1995. Calcium imaging of single stereocilia in hair cells: localization of transduction channels at both ends of tip links. Neuron 15, 1311–1321.

Densert, O., Flock, A. 1974. An electron-microscopic study of adrenergic innervation in the cochlea. Acta Otolaryngol 77, 185–197.

Dewson, J.H. 1968. Efferent olivocochlear bundle: some relationships to stimulus discrimination in noise. J Neurophysiol 31, 122–130.

van Dijk, P., Wit, H.P., Segenhout, J.M., Tubis, A. 1994. Wiener kernel analysis of inner ear function in the American bullfrog. J Acoust Soc Am 95, 904–919.

Dolan, D.F., Guo, M.H., Nuttall, A.L. 1997. Frequency-dependent enhancement of basilar membrane velocity during olivocochlear bundle stimulation. J Acoust Soc Am 102, 3587–3596.

Donaudy, F., Zheng, L., Ficarella, R., Ballana, E., Carella, M., Melchionda, S., Estivill, X., Bartles, J.R., Gasparini, P. 2006. Espin gene (ESPN) mutations associated with autosomal dominant hearing loss cause defects in microvillar elongation or organisation. J Med Genet 43, 157–161.

Dorsaint-Pierre, R., Penhune, V.B., Watkins, K.E., Neelin, P., Lerch, J.P., Bouffard, M., Zatorre, R.J. 2006. Asymmetries of the planum temporale and Heschl's gyrus: relationship to language lateralization. Brain 129, 1164–1176.

Doucet, J.R., Ryugo, D.K. 1997. Projections from the ventral cochlear nucleus to the dorsal cochlear nucleus in rats. J Comp Neurol 385, 245–264.

Doucet, J.R., Ryugo, D.K. 2003. Axonal pathways to the lateral superior olive labeled with biotinylated dextran amine injections in the dorsal cochlear nucleus of rats. J Comp Neurol 461, 452–465.

Drenckhahn, D., Schafer, T., Prinz, M. 1985. Actin, myosin and associated proteins in the auditory and vestibular organs: immunocytochemical and biochemical studies. In: Drescher, D.G. (Ed.), Auditory Biochemistry. Thomas, Springfield. pp. 436–472.

Dronkers, N.F., Wilkins, D.P., Van Valin, R.D., Jr., Redfern, B.B., Jaeger, J.J. 2004. Lesion analysis of the brain areas involved in language comprehension. Cognition 92, 145–177.

Dumont, R.A., Zhao, Y.D., Holt, J.R., Bahler, M., Gillespie, P.G. 2002. Myosin-I isozymes in neonatal rodent auditory and vestibular epithelia. J Assoc Res Otolaryngol 3, 375–389.

Durlach, N.I. 1972. Binaural signal detection: equalization and cancellation theory. In: Tobias, J.V. (Ed.), Foundations of Modern Auditory Theory, Vol. 2. Academic Press, New York.

Duvel, A.D., Smith, D.M., Talk, A., Gabriel, M. 2001. Medial geniculate, amygdalar and cingulate cortical training-induced neuronal activity during discriminative avoidance learning in rabbits with auditory cortical lesions. J Neurosci 21, 3271–3281.

Edeline, J.M., Weinberger, N.M. 1991. Subcortical adaptive filtering in the auditory system: associative receptive field plasticity in the dorsal medial geniculate body. Behav Neurosci 105, 154–175.

Edeline, J.M., Manunta, Y., Nodal, F.R., Bajo, V.M. 1999. Do auditory responses recorded from awake animals reflect the anatomical parcellation of the auditory thalamus? Hear Res 131, 135–152.

Egan, J.P., Hake, H.W. 1950. On the masking pattern of a simple auditory stimulus. J Acoust Soc Am 22, 622–630.

Eggermont, J.J. 2005. Tinnitus: neurobiological substrates. Drug Discov Today 10, 1283–1290.

Eldredge, D.H. 1974. Inner ear-cochlear mechanics and cochlear potentials. In: Keidel, W.D., Neff, W.D. (Eds), Handbook of Sensory Physiology, Vol. 5/1. Springer, Berlin. pp. 549–584.

Elgoyhen, A.B., Vetter, D.E., Katz, E., Rothlin, C.V., Heinemann, S.F., Boulter, J. 2001. Alpha10: a determinant of nicotinic cholinergic receptor function in mammalian vestibular and cochlear mechanosensory hair cells. Proc Natl Acad Sci USA 98, 3501–3506.

Elliott, D.N., Stein, L., Harrison, M.J. 1960. Discrimination of absolute-intensity thresholds and frequency-difference thresholds in cats. J Acoust Soc Am 32, 380–384.

Elverland, H.H. 1977. Descending connections between superior olivary and cochlear nuclear complexes in the cat studied by autoradiographic and horseradish peroxidase methods. Exp Brain Res 27, 397–412.

Elverland, H.H. 1978. Ascending and intrinsic projections of the superior olivary complex in the cat. Exp Brain Res 32, 117–134.

Emadi, G., Richter, C.P., Dallos, P. 2004. Stiffness of the gerbil basilar membrane: radial and longitudinal variations. J Neurophysiol 91, 474–488.

Escabi, M.A., Schreiner, C.E. 2002. Nonlinear spectrotemporal sound analysis by neurons in the auditory midbrain. J Neurosci 22, 4114–4131.

Evans, E.F. 1972. The frequency response and other properties of single fibres in the guinea-pig cochlear nerve. J Physiol 226, 263–287.

Evans, E.F. 1975. Cochlear nerve and cochlear nucleus. In: Keidel, W.D., Neff, W.D. (Eds), Handbook of Sensory Physiology, Vol. 5/2. Springer, Berlin. pp. 1–108.

Evans, E.F. 1977. Frequency selectivity at high signal levels of single units in cochlear nerve and nucleus. In: Evans, E.F., Wilson, J.P. (Eds), Psychophysics and Physiology of Hearing. Academic Press, London. pp. 185–192.

Evans, E.F., Harrison, R.V. 1976. Proceedings: Correlation between cochlear outer hair cell damage and deterioration of cochlear nerve tuning properties in the guinea-pig. J Physiol 256, 43P–44P.

Evans, E.F., Nelson, P.G. 1973. The responses of single neurones in the cochlear nucleus of the cat as a function of their location and the anaesthetic state. Exp Brain Res 17, 402–427.

Eybalin, M. 1993. Neurotransmitters and neuromodulators of the mammalian cochlea. Physiol Rev 73, 309–373.

Faingold, C.L. 1999. Neuronal networks in the genetically epilepsy-prone rat. Adv Neurol 79, 311–321.

Farris, H.E., LeBlanc, C.L., Goswami, J., Ricci, A.J. 2004. Probing the pore of the auditory hair cell mechanotransducer channel in turtle. J Physiol 558, 769–792.

Fauser, C., Schimanski, S., Wangemann, P. 2004. Localization of beta1-adrenergic receptors in the cochlea and the vestibular labyrinth. J Membr Biol 201, 25–32.

Fawcett, D.W. 1986. A Textbook of Histology. W.B. Saunders, Philadelphia.

Felix, H. 2002. Anatomical differences in the peripheral auditory system of mammals and man. A mini review. Adv Otorhinolaryngol 59, 1–10.

Felix, D., Ehrenberger, K. 1992. The efferent modulation of mammalian inner hair cell afferents. Hear Res 64, 1–5.

Ferragamo, M.J., Oertel, D. 2002. Octopus cells of the mammalian ventral cochlear nucleus sense the rate of depolarization. J Neurophysiol 87, 2262–2270.

Fettiplace, R. 2006. Active hair bundle movements in auditory hair cells. J Physiol 576, 29–36.

Fettiplace, R., Ricci, A.J. 2003. Adaptation in auditory hair cells. Curr Opin Neurobiol 13, 446–451.

Finsterer, J., Fellinger, J. 2005. Nuclear and mitochondrial genes mutated in nonsyndromic impaired hearing. Int J Pediatr Otorhinolaryngol 69, 621–647.

Firszt, J.B., Ulmer, J.L., Gaggl, W. 2006. Differential representation of speech sounds in the human cerebral hemispheres. Anat Rec A Discov Mol Cell Evol Biol 288, 345–357.

Fischel-Ghodsian, N., Kopke, R.D., Ge, X. 2004. Mitochondrial dysfunction in hearing loss. Mitochondrion 4, 675–694.

Fletcher, H. 1940. Auditory patterns. Rev Mod Phys 12, 47–65.

Flock, A., Flock, B., Murray, E. 1977. Studies on the sensory hairs of receptor cells in the inner ear. Acta Otolaryngol 83, 85–91.

Flock, A., Bretscher, A., Weber, K. 1982. Immunohistochemical localization of several cytoskeletal proteins in inner ear sensory and supporting cells. Hear Res 7, 75–89.

Forge, A., Li, L. 2000. Apoptotic death of hair cells in mammalian vestibular sensory epithelia. Hear Res 139, 97–115.

Forge, A., Schacht, J. 2000. Aminoglycoside antibiotics. Audiol Neurootol 5, 3–22.

Forge, A., Van De Water, T.R. 2008. Protection and repair of inner ear sensory cells. In: Salvi, R.J., Popper, A.N., Fay, R.R. (Eds), Regeneration and Repair. Springer Handbook of Auditory Research, Vol. 33. Springer, New York.

Forge, A., Li, L., Corwin, J.T., Nevill, G. 1993. Ultrastructural evidence for hair cell regeneration in the mammalian inner ear. Science 259, 1616–1619.

Formisano, E., Kim, D.S., Di Salle, F., van de Moortele, P.F., Ugurbil, K., Goebel, R. 2003. Mirror-symmetric tonotopic maps in human primary auditory cortex. Neuron 40, 859–869.

Friauf, E., Hammerschmidt, B., Kirsch, J. 1997. Development of adult-type inhibitory glycine receptors in the central auditory system of rats. J Comp Neurol 385, 117–134.

Fridberger, A., de Monvel, J.B., Zheng, J., Hu, N., Zou, Y., Ren, T., Nuttall, A. 2004. Organ of Corti potentials and the motion of the basilar membrane. J Neurosci 24, 10057–10063.

Frisina, R.D. 2001. Subcortical neural coding mechanisms for auditory temporal processing. Hear Res 158, 1–27.

Fritz, J., Shamma, S., Elhilali, M., Klein, D. 2003. Rapid task-related plasticity of spectrotemporal receptive fields in primary auditory cortex. Nat Neurosci 6, 1216–1223.

Frohne, C., Lesinski, A., Battmer, R.D., Lenarz, T. 1997. Intraoperative test of auditory nerve function. Am J Otol 18, S93–S94.

Fujino, K., Oertel, D. 2001. Cholinergic modulation of stellate cells in the mammalian ventral cochlear nucleus. J Neurosci 21, 7372–7383.

Gagnaire, F., Langlais, C. 2005. Relative ototoxicity of 21 aromatic solvents. Arch Toxicol 79, 346–354.

Galaburda, A., Sanides, F. 1980. Cytoarchitectonic organization of the human auditory cortex. J Comp Neurol 190, 597–610.

Gates, G.A., Couropmitree, N.N., Myers, R.H. 1999. Genetic associations in age-related hearing thresholds. Arch Otolaryngol Head Neck Surg 125, 654–659.

Geers, A.E. 2004. Speech, language, and reading skills after early cochlear implantation. Arch Otolaryngol Head Neck Surg 130, 634–648.

Geisler, C.D., Nuttall, A.L. 1997. Two-tone suppression of basilar membrane vibrations in the base of the guinea pig cochlea using "low-side" suppressors. J Acoust Soc Am 102, 430–440.

Geleoc, G.S., Lennan, G.W., Richardson, G.P., Kros, C.J. 1997. A quantitative comparison of mechanoelectrical transduction in vestibular and auditory hair cells of neonatal mice. Proc Roy Soc Biol Sci 264, 611–621.

Geschwind, N., Levitsky, W. 1968. Human brain: left-right asymmetries in temporal speech region. Science 161, 186–187.

Gilbert, A.G., Pickles, J.O. 1980. Responses of auditory nerve fibres in the guinea pig to noise bands of different widths. Hear Res 2, 327–333.

Gillespie, P.G. 2004. Myosin I and adaptation of mechanical transduction by the inner ear. Philos Trans R Soc Lond B Biol Sci 359, 1945–1951.

Gillespie, L.N., Shepherd, R.K. 2005. Clinical application of neurotrophic factors: the potential for primary auditory neuron protection. Eur J Neurosci 22, 2123–2133.

Gillespie, P.G., Dumont, R.A., Kachar, B. 2005. Have we found the tip link, transduction channel, and gating spring of the hair cell? Curr Opin Neurobiol 15, 389–396.

Giraud, A.L., Garnier, S., Micheyl, C., Lina, G., Chays, A., Chery-Croze, S. 1997. Auditory efferents involved in speech-in-noise intelligibility. Neuroreport 8, 1779–1783.

Girod, D.A., Rubel, E.W. 1991. Hair cell regeneration in the avian cochlea: if it works in birds, why not in man? Ear Nose Throat J 70, 343–350, 353–354.

Girod, D.A., Duckert, L.G., Rubel, E.W. 1989. Possible precursors of regenerated hair cells in the avian cochlea following acoustic trauma. Hear Res 42, 175–194.

Glendenning, K.K., Baker, B.N., Hutson, K.A., Masterton, R.B. 1992. Acoustic chiasm V: inhibition and excitation in the ipsilateral and contralateral projections of LSO. J Comp Neurol 319, 100–122.

Glueckert, R., Pfaller, K., Kinnefors, A., Schrott-Fischer, A., Rask-Andersen, H. 2005. High resolution scanning electron microscopy of the human organ of Corti. A study using freshly fixed surgical specimens. Hear Res 199, 40–56.

Goblick, T.J., Jr., Pfeiffer, R.R. 1969. Time-domain measurements of cochlear nonlinearities using combination click stimuli. J Acoust Soc Am 46, 924–938.

Goldberg, J.M., Brown, P.B. 1969. Response of binaural neurons of dog superior olivary complex to dichotic tonal stimuli: some physiological mechanisms of sound localization. J Neurophysiol 32, 613–636.

Goldberg, J.M., Brownell, W.E. 1973. Discharge characteristics of neurons in anteroventral and dorsal cochlear nuclei of cat. Brain Res 64, 35–54.

Goldstein, J.L. 1967. Auditory nonlinearity. J Acoust Soc Am 41, 676–689.

Goldstein, J.L., Kiang, N.Y.S. 1968. Neural correlates of the aural combination tone $2f_1 - f_2$. Proc IEEE 56, 981–992.

Goodyear, R.J., Richardson, G.P. 2002. Extracellular matrices associated with the apical surfaces of sensory epithelia in the inner ear: molecular and structural diversity. J Neurobiol 53, 212–227.

Gourevitch, B., Eggermont, J.J. 2007. Spatial representation of neural responses to natural and altered conspecific vocalizations in cat auditory cortex. J Neurophysiol 97, 144–158.

Gow, A., Davies, C., Southwood, C.M., Frolenkov, G., Chrustowski, M., Ng, L., Yamauchi, D., Marcus, D.C., Kachar, B. 2004. Deafness in Claudin 11-null mice reveals the critical contribution of basal cell tight junctions to stria vascularis function. J Neurosci 24, 7051–7062.

Greenwood, D.D., Goldberg, J.M. 1970. Response of neurons in the cochlear nuclei to variations in noise bandwidth and to tone-noise combinations. J Acoust Soc Am 47, 1022–1040.

Griffiths, T.D., Warren, J.D. 2002. The planum temporale as a computational hub. Trends Neurosci 25, 348–353.

Groff, J.A., Liberman, M.C. 2003. Modulation of cochlear afferent response by the lateral olivocochlear system: activation via electrical stimulation of the inferior colliculus. J Neurophysiol 90, 3178–3200.

Grosh, K., Zheng, J., Zou, Y., de Boer, E., Nuttall, A.L. 2004. High-frequency electromotile responses in the cochlea. J Acoust Soc Am 115, 2178–2184.

Grothe, B., Sanes, D.H. 1993. Bilateral inhibition by glycinergic afferents in the medial superior olive. J Neurophysiol 69, 1192–1196.

Howard, J., Roberts, W.M., Hudspeth, A.J. 1988. Mechanoelectrical transduction by hair cells. Annu Rev Biophys Biophys Chem 17, 99–124.

Huang, C.L., Larue, D.T., Winer, J.A. 1999. GABAergic organization of the cat medial geniculate body. J Comp Neurol 415, 368–392.

Hubbard, A.E., Mountain, D.C. 1996. Analysis and synthesis of cochlear mechanical models. In: Hawkins, H.L., McMullen, T.A., Popper, A.N., Fay, R.R. (Eds), Auditory Computation, Springer Handbook of Auditory Research, Vol. 6. Springer, New York. pp. 62–120.

Hubel, D.H., Wiesel, T.N. 1962. Receptive fields, binocular interaction and functional architecture in the cat's visual cortex. J Physiol 160, 106–154.

Hudspeth, A.J., Corey, D.P. 1977. Sensitivity, polarity, and conductance change in the response of vertebrate hair cells to controlled mechanical stimuli. Proc Natl Acad Sci USA 74, 2407–2411.

Hudspeth, A.J., Jacobs, R. 1979. Stereocilia mediate transduction in vertebrate hair cells. Proc Natl Acad Sci USA 76, 1506–1509.

Hutchin, T.P., Cortopassi, G.A. 2000. Mitochondrial defects and hearing loss. Cell Mol Life Sci 57, 1927–1937.

Ikeda, K., Oshima, T., Hidaka, H., Takasaka, T. 1997. Molecular and clinical implications of loop diuretic ototoxicity. Hear Res 107, 1–8.

Imaizumi, K., Priebe, N.J., Crum, P.A., Bedenbaugh, P.H., Cheung, S.W., Schreiner, C.E. 2004. Modular functional organization of cat anterior auditory field. J Neurophysiol 92, 444–457.

Imig, T.J., Adrian, H.O. 1977. Binaural columns in the primary field (A1) of cat auditory cortex. Brain Res 138, 241–257.

Imig, T.J., Brugge, J.F. 1978. Sources and terminations of callosal axons related to binaural and frequency maps in primary auditory cortex of the cat. J Comp Neurol 182, 637–660.

Indefrey, P., Levelt, W.J. 2004. The spatial and temporal signatures of word production components. Cognition 92, 101–144.

Ingham, N.J., McAlpine, D. 2005. GABAergic inhibition controls neural gain in inferior colliculus neurons sensitive to interaural time differences. J Neurosci 25, 6187–6198.

Irvine, D.R.F. 1986. The auditory brainstem. Prog Sens Physiol 7, 1–279.

Irvine, D.R., Rajan, R., Aitkin, L.M. 1996. Sensitivity to interaural intensity differences of neurons in primary auditory cortex of the cat. I. Types of sensitivity and effects of variations in sound pressure level. J Neurophysiol 75, 75–96.

Ito, M., van Adel, B., Kelly, J.B. 1996. Sound localization after transection of the commissure of Probst in the albino rat. J Neurophysiol 76, 3493–3502.

Izumikawa, M., Minoda, R., Kawamoto, K., Abrashkin, K.A., Swiderski, D.L., Dolan, D.F., Brough, D.E., Raphael, Y. 2005. Auditory hair cell replacement and hearing improvement by Atoh1 gene therapy in deaf mammals. Nat Med 11, 271–276.

Jain, R., Shore, S. 2006. External inferior colliculus integrates trigeminal and acoustic information: unit responses to trigeminal nucleus and acoustic stimulation in the guinea pig. Neurosci Lett 395, 71–75.

Jastreboff, P.J., Jastreboff, M.M. 2006. Tinnitus retraining therapy: a different view on tinnitus. ORL J Otorhinolaryngol Relat Spec 68, 23–29; discussion 29–30.

Jastreboff, P.J., Brennan, J.F., Coleman, J.K., Sasaki, C.T. 1988. Phantom auditory sensation in rats: an animal model for tinnitus. Behav Neurosci 102, 811–822.

Javel, E., Shepherd, R.K. 2000. Electrical stimulation of the auditory nerve. III. Response initiation sites and temporal fine structure. Hear Res 140, 45–76.

Javel, E., McGee, J., Walsh, E.J., Farley, G.R., Gorga, M.P. 1983. Suppression of auditory nerve responses. II. Suppression threshold and growth, iso-suppression contours. J Acoust Soc Am 74, 801–813.

Jeffress, L.A. 1948. A place theory of sound localization. J Comp Physiol Psychol 41, 35–39.

Jen, P.H., Chen, Q.C., Wu, F.J. 2002. Interaction between excitation and inhibition affects frequency tuning curve, response size and latency of neurons in the auditory cortex of the big brown bat, *Eptesicus fuscus*. Hear Res 174, 281–289.

Jenkins, W.M., Masterton, R.B. 1982. Sound localization: effects of unilateral lesions in central auditory system. J Neurophysiol 47, 987–1016.

Jenkins, W.M., Merzenich, M.M. 1984. Role of cat primary auditory cortex for sound-localization behavior. J Neurophysiol 52, 819–847.

Jia, S., He, D.Z. 2005. Motility-associated hair-bundle motion in mammalian outer hair cells. Nat Neurosci 8, 1028–1034.

Jia, S., Dallos, P., He, D.Z. 2007. Mechanoelectric transduction of adult inner hair cells. J Neurosci 27, 1006–1014.

Jiang, D., McAlpine, D., Palmer, A.R. 1997. Detectability index measures of binaural masking level difference across populations of inferior colliculus neurons. J Neurosci 17, 9331–9339.

Jiang, H., Sha, S.H., Forge, A., Schacht, J. 2006. Caspase-independent pathways of hair cell death induced by kanamycin in vivo. Cell Death Differ 13, 20–30.

Johnstone, B.M., Sellick, P.M. 1972. The peripheral auditory apparatus. Q Rev Biophys 5, 1–57.

Johnstone, B.M., Patuzzi, R., Yates, G.K. 1986. Basilar membrane measurements and the travelling wave. Hear Res 22, 147–153.

Johnstone, B.M., Patuzzi, R., Syka, J., Sykova, E. 1989. Stimulus-related potassium changes in the organ of Corti of guinea-pig. J Physiol 408, 77–92.

Joris, P.X. 1998. Response classes in the dorsal cochlear nucleus and its output tract in the chloralose-anesthetized cat. J Neurosci 18, 3955–3966.

Joris, P.X., Yin, T.C. 1998. Envelope coding in the lateral superior olive. III. Comparison with afferent pathways. J Neurophysiol 79, 253–269.

Joris, P., Yin, T.C. 2007. A matter of time: internal delays in binaural processing. Trends Neurosci 30, 70–78.

Joris, P.X., Carney, L.H., Smith, P.H., Yin, T.C. 1994a. Enhancement of neural synchronization in the anteroventral cochlear nucleus. I. Responses to tones at the characteristic frequency. J Neurophysiol 71, 1022–1036.

Joris, P.X., Smith, P.H., Yin, T.C. 1994b. Enhancement of neural synchronization in the anteroventral cochlear nucleus. II. Responses in the tuning curve tail. J Neurophysiol 71, 1037–1051.

Joris, P.X., Schreiner, C.E., Rees, A. 2004. Neural processing of amplitude-modulated sounds. Physiol Rev 84, 541–577.

Kaas, J.H., Hackett, T.A. 2000. Subdivisions of auditory cortex and processing streams in primates. Proc Natl Acad Sci USA 97, 11793–11799.

Kachar, B., Parakkal, M., Kurc, M., Zhao, Y., Gillespie, P.G. 2000. High-resolution structure of hair-cell tip links. Proc Natl Acad Sci USA 97, 13336–13341.

Kadia, S.C., Wang, X. 2003. Spectral integration in A1 of awake primates: neurons with single- and multipeaked tuning characteristics. J Neurophysiol 89, 1603–1622.

Kajikawa, Y., de La Mothe, L., Blumell, S., Hackett, T.A. 2005. A comparison of neuron response properties in areas A1 and CM of the marmoset monkey auditory cortex: tones and broadband noise. J Neurophysiol 93, 22–34.

Kaltenbach, J.A. 2006. The dorsal cochlear nucleus as a participant in the auditory, attentional and emotional components of tinnitus. Hear Res 216–217, 224–234.

Kaltenbach, J.A., Godfrey, D.A., Neumann, J.B., McCaslin, D.L., Afman, C.E., Zhang, J. 1998. Changes in spontaneous neural activity in the dorsal cochlear nucleus following exposure to intense sound: relation to threshold shift. Hear Res 124, 78–84.

Kaltenbach, J.A., Rachel, J.D., Mathog, T.A., Zhang, J., Falzarano, P.R., Lewandowski, M. 2002. Cisplatin-induced hyperactivity in the dorsal cochlear nucleus and its relation to outer hair cell loss: relevance to tinnitus. J Neurophysiol 88, 699–714.

Kanwal, J.S., Fitzpatrick, D.C., Suga, N. 1999. Facilitatory and inhibitory frequency tuning of combination-sensitive neurons in the primary auditory cortex of mustached bats. J Neurophysiol 82, 2327–2345.

Kanzaki, S., Beyer, L.A., Swiderski, D.L., Izumikawa, M., Stover, T., Kawamoto, K., Raphael, Y. 2006a. p27(Kip1) deficiency causes organ of Corti pathology and hearing loss. Hear Res 214, 28–36.

Kanzaki, S., Beyer, L., Karolyi, I.J., Dolan, D.F., Fang, Q., Probst, F.J., Camper, S.A., Raphael, Y. 2006b. Transgene correction maintains normal cochlear structure and function in 6-month-old Myo15a mutant mice. Hear Res 214, 37–44.

Kavanagh, G.L., Kelly, J.B. 1987. Contribution of auditory cortex to sound localization by the ferret (Mustela putorius). J Neurophysiol 57, 1746–1766.

Kawamoto, K., Ishimoto, S., Minoda, R., Brough, D.E., Raphael, Y. 2003. Math1 gene transfer generates new cochlear hair cells in mature guinea pigs in vivo. J Neurosci 23, 4395–4400.

Kawase, T., Delgutte, B., Liberman, M.C. 1993. Antimasking effects of the olivocochlear reflex. II. Enhancement of auditory-nerve response to masked tones. J Neurophysiol 70, 2533–2549.

Kazmierczak, P., Sakaguchi, H., Tokita, J., Wilson-Kubalek, E.M., Milligan, R.A., Muller, U., Kachar, B. 2007. Cadherin 23 and protocadherin 15 interact to form tip-link filaments in sensory hair cells. Nature 449, 87–91.

Kelley, M.W. 2006. Regulation of cell fate in the sensory epithelia of the inner ear. Nat Rev Neurosci 7, 837–849.

Kelly, J.B. 1997. Contributions of the dorsal nucleus of the lateral lemnsicus to binaural processing in the auditory brainstem. In: Syka, J. (Ed.), Acoustical Signal Processing in the Central Auditory System. Plenum, New York. pp. 329–352.

Kelly, J.B., Li, L., van Adel, B. 1996. Sound localization after kainic acid lesions of the dorsal nucleus of the lateral lemniscus in the albino rat. Behav Neurosci 110, 1445–1455.

Kemp, D.T. 1978. Stimulated acoustic emissions from within the human auditory system. J Acoust Soc Am 64, 1386–1391.

Kemp, D.T. 2002. Otoacoustic emissions, their origin in cochlear function, and use. Br Med Bull 63, 223–241.

Kennedy, H.J., Evans, M.G., Crawford, A.C., Fettiplace, R. 2003. Fast adaptation of mechanoelectrical transducer channels in mammalian cochlear hair cells. Nat Neurosci 6, 832–836.

Kennedy, H.J., Crawford, A.C., Fettiplace, R. 2005. Force generation by mammalian hair bundles supports a role in cochlear amplification. Nature 433, 880–883.

Kennedy, H.J., Evans, M.G., Crawford, A.C., Fettiplace, R. 2006. Depolarization of cochlear outer hair cells evokes active hair bundle motion by two mechanisms. J Neurosci 26, 2757–2766.

Kessel, R.G., Kardon, R.H. 1979. Tissues and Organs. W.H. Freeman and Company, San Fransisco.

Khalfa, S., Bougeard, R., Morand, N., Veuillet, E., Isnard, J., Guenot, M., Ryvlin, P., Fischer, C., Collet, L. 2001. Evidence of peripheral auditory activity modulation by the auditory cortex in humans. Neuroscience 104, 347–358.

Khanna, S.M., Tonndorf, J. 1972. Tympanic membrane vibrations in cats studied by time-averaged holography. J Acoust Soc Am 51, 1904–1920.

Kiang, N.Y. 1980. Processing of speech by the auditory nervous system. J Acoust Soc Am 68, 830–835.

Kiang, N.Y. 1990. Curious oddments of auditory-nerve studies. Hear Res 49, 1–16.

Kiang, N.Y., Moxon, E.C. 1972. Physiological considerations in artificial stimulation of the inner ear. Ann Otol Rhinol Laryngol 81, 714–730.

Kiang, N.Y., Watanabe, T., Thomas, E.C., Clark, L.F. 1962. Stimulus coding in the cat's auditory nerve. Preliminary report. Ann Otol Rhinol Laryngol 71, 1009–1026.

Kiang, N.Y.S., Watanabe, T., Thomas, E.C., Clark, L.F. 1965. Discharge Patterns of Single Fibers in the Cat's Auditory Nerve MIT Press, Cambridge.

Kiang, N.Y., Sachs, M.B., Peake, W.T. 1967. Shapes of tuning curves for single auditory-nerve fibers. J Acoust Soc Am 42, 1341–1342.

Kiang, N.Y., Moxon, E.C., Levine, R.A. 1970. Auditory-nerve activity in cats with normal and abnormal cochleas. In: Sensorineural hearing loss. Ciba Found Symp, 241–273.

Kidd, S.A., Kelly, J.B. 1996. Contribution of the dorsal nucleus of the lateral lemniscus to binaural responses in the inferior colliculus of the rat: interaural time delays. J Neurosci 16, 7390–7397.

Kim, D.O., Molnar, C.E., Matthews, J.W. 1980. Cochlear mechanics: nonlinear behavior in two-tone responses as reflected in cochlear-nerve-fiber responses and in ear-canal sound pressure. J Acoust Soc Am 67, 1704–1721.

Kim, D.O., Sirianni, J.G., Chang, S.O. 1990. Responses of DCN-PVCN neurons and auditory nerve fibers in unanesthetized decerebrate cats to AM and pure tones: analysis with autocorrelation/power-spectrum. Hear Res 45, 95–113.

Kittel, M., Wagner, E., Klump, G.M. 2002. An estimate of the auditory-filter bandwidth in the Mongolian gerbil. Hear Res 164, 69–76.

Kluk, K., Moore, B.C. 2005. Factors affecting psychophysical tuning curves for hearing-impaired subjects with high-frequency dead regions. Hear Res 200, 115–131.

Knudsen, E.I., Konishi, M. 1978. A neural map of auditory space in the owl. Science 200, 795–797.

Koch, M. 1999. The neurobiology of startle. Prog Neurobiol 59, 107–128.

Koch, U., Grothe, B. 2003. Hyperpolarization-activated current (Ih) in the inferior colliculus: distribution and contribution to temporal processing. J Neurophysiol 90, 3679–3687.

Koike, T., Wada, H., Kobayashi, T. 2002. Modeling of the human middle ear using the finite-element method. J Acoust Soc Am 111, 1306–1317.

Kopp-Scheinpflug, C., Dehmel, S., Dorrscheidt, G.J., Rübsamen, R. 2002. Interaction of excitation and inhibition in anteroventral cochlear nucleus neurons that receive large endbulb synaptic endings. J Neurosci 22, 11004–11018.

Kopp-Scheinpflug, C., Lippe, W.R., Dorrscheidt, G.J., Rübsamen, R. 2003. The medial nucleus of the trapezoid body in the gerbil is more than a relay: comparison of pre- and postsynaptic activity. J Assoc Res Otolaryngol 4, 1–23.

Kringlebotn, M. 1988. Network model for the human middle ear. Scand Audiol 17, 75–85.

Krishna, B.S., Semple, M.N. 2000. Auditory temporal processing: responses to sinusoidally amplitude-modulated tones in the inferior colliculus. J Neurophysiol 84, 255–273.

Kromer, L.F., Moore, R.Y. 1980. Norepinephrine innervation of the cochlear nuclei by locus coeruleus neurons in the rat. Anat Embryol (Berl) 158, 227–244.

Kros, C.J. 1996. Physiology of mammalian cochlear hair cells. In: Dallos, P., Popper, A.N., Fay, R.R. (Eds), The Cochlea, Springer Handbook of Auditory Research, Vol. 8. Springer, New York. pp. 318–385.

Kros, C.J. 2007. How to build an inner hair cell: challenges for regeneration. Hear Res 227, 3–10

Kros, C.J., Rüsch, A., Richardson, G.P. 1992. Mechano-electrical transducer currents in hair cells of the cultured neonatal mouse cochlea. Proc Roy Soc Biol Sci 249, 185–193.

Krumbholz, K., Schonwiesner, M., von Cramon, D.Y., Rubsamen, R., Shah, N.J., Zilles, K., Fink, G.R. 2005. Representation of interaural temporal information from left and right auditory space in the human planum temporale and inferior parietal lobe. Cereb Cortex 15, 317–324.

Kuhl, P.K. 2004. Early language acquisition: cracking the speech code. Nat Rev Neurosci 5, 831–843.

Kuijpers, W., Bonting, S.L. 1969. Studies on (Na^+-K^+)-activated ATPase. XXIV. Localization and properties of ATPase in the inner ear of the guinea pig. Biochim Biophys Acta 173, 477–485.

Kuijpers, W., Bonting, S.L. 1970. The cochlear potentials. I. The effect of ouabain on the cochlear potentials of the guinea pig. Pflugers Arch 320, 348–358.

Kujawa, S.G., Liberman, M.C. 1997. Conditioning-related protection from acoustic injury: effects of chronic deefferentation and sham surgery. J Neurophysiol 78, 3095–3106.

Kumar, S., Stephan, K.E., Warren, J.D., Friston, K.J., Griffiths, T.D. 2007. Hierarchical Processing of Auditory Objects in Humans. PLoS Comput Biol 3, e100. Epub 2007 Apr 24.

Kummer, P., Janssen, T., Arnold, W. 1995. Suppression tuning characteristics of the $2f_1-f_2$ distortion-product otoacoustic emission in humans. J Acoust Soc Am 98, 197–210.

Kuwada, S., Fitzpatrick, D.C., Batra, R., Ostapoff, E.M. 2006. Sensitivity to interaural time differences in the dorsal nucleus of the lateral lemniscus of the unanesthetized rabbit: comparison with other structures. J Neurophysiol 95, 1309–1322.

Kwan, K.Y., Allchorne, A.J., Vollrath, M.A., Christensen, A.P., Zhang, D.S., Woolf, C.J., Corey, D.P. 2006. TRPA1 contributes to cold, mechanical, and chemical nociception but is not essential for hair-cell transduction. Neuron 50, 277–289.

Kwon, J., Pierson, M. 1997. Fos-immunoreactive responses in inferior colliculi of rats with experimental audiogenic seizure susceptibility. Epilepsy Res 27, 89–99.

Lane, C.C., Delgutte, B. 2005. Neural correlates and mechanisms of spatial release from masking: single-unit and population responses in the inferior colliculus. J Neurophysiol 94, 1180–1198.

Langner, G. 2004. Topographic representation of periodicity information: the 2nd neural axis of the auditory system. In: Syka, J., Merzenich, M.M. (Eds), Plasticity of the Central Auditory System and Processing of Complex Acoustic Signals. Plenum, New York. pp. 19–33.

Langner, G. 2005. Neuronal mechanisms underlying the perception of pitch and harmony. Ann N Y Acad Sci 1060, 50–52.

Langner, G., Schreiner, C.E. 1988. Periodicity coding in the inferior colliculus of the cat. I. Neuronal mechanisms. J Neurophysiol 60, 1799–1822.

Langner, G., Albert, M., Briede, T. 2002. Temporal and spatial coding of periodicity information in the inferior colliculus of awake chinchilla (Chinchilla laniger). Hear Res 168, 110–130.

Laroche, C., Hetu, R., Quoc, H.T., Josserand, B., Glasberg, B. 1992. Frequency selectivity in workers with noise-induced hearing loss. Hear Res 64, 61–72.

Leake, P.A., Rebscher, S.J. 2004. Anatomical considerations and long-term effects of electrical stimulation. In: Zeng, F.G., Popper, A.N., Fay, R.R. (Eds), Cochlear Implants: Auditory Prostheses and Electric Hearing, Springer Handbook of Auditory Research, Vol. 20. Springer, New York. pp. 101–148.

LeBeau, F.E., Malmierca, M.S., Rees, A. 2001. Iontophoresis in vivo demonstrates a key role for GABA(A) and glycinergic inhibition in shaping frequency response areas in the inferior colliculus of guinea pig. J Neurosci 21, 7303–7312.

LeDoux, J.E., Cicchetti, P., Xagoraris, A., Romanski, L.M. 1990. The lateral amygdaloid nucleus: sensory interface of the amygdala in fear conditioning. J Neurosci 10, 1062–1069.

Lee, A., Kannan, V., Hillis, A.E. 2006. The contribution of neuroimaging to the study of language and aphasia. Neuropsychol Rev 16, 171–183.

Legan, P.K., Rau, A., Keen, J.N., Richardson, G.P. 1997. The mouse tectorins. Modular matrix proteins of the inner ear homologous to components of the sperm-egg adhesion system. J Biol Chem 272, 8791–8801.

LeMasurier, M., Gillespie, P.G. 2005. Hair-cell mechanotransduction and cochlear amplification. Neuron 48, 403–415.

Lesniak, W., Pecoraro, V.L., Schacht, J. 2005. Ternary complexes of gentamicin with iron and lipid catalyze formation of reactive oxygen species. Chem Res Toxicol 18, 357–364.

Li, L., Forge, A. 1997. Morphological evidence for supporting cell to hair cell conversion in the mammalian utricular macula. Int J Dev Neurosci 15, 433–446.

Li, L., Kelly, J.B. 1992. Inhibitory influence of the dorsal nucleus of the lateral lemniscus on binaural responses in the rat's inferior colliculus. J Neurosci 12, 4530–459.

Li, H., Roblin, G., Liu, H., Heller, S. 2003. Generation of hair cells by stepwise differentiation of embryonic stem cells. Proc Natl Acad Sci USA 100, 13495–13500.

Liberman, M.C. 1978. Auditory-nerve response from cats raised in a low-noise chamber. J Acoust Soc Am 63, 442–455.

Liberman, M.C. 1980. Efferent synapses in the inner hair cell area of the cat cochlea: an electron microscopic study of serial sections. Hear Res 3, 189–204.

Liberman, M.C. 1982. Single-neuron labeling in the cat auditory nerve. Science 216, 1239–1241.

Liberman, M.C., Dodds, L.W. 1984a. Single-neuron labeling and chronic cochlear pathology. II. Stereocilia damage and alterations of spontaneous discharge rates. Hear Res 16, 43–53.

Liberman, M.C., Dodds, L.W. 1984b. Single-neuron labeling and chronic cochlear pathology. III. Stereocilia damage and alterations of threshold tuning curves. Hear Res 16, 55–74.

Liberman, M.C., Dodds, L.W. 1987. Acute ultrastructural changes in acoustic trauma: serial-section reconstruction of stereocilia and cuticular plates. Hear Res 26, 45–64.

Liberman, M.C., Kiang, N.Y. 1978. Acoustic trauma in cats. Cochlear pathology and auditory-nerve activity. Acta Otolaryngol Suppl 358, 1–63.

Liberman, A.M., Cooper, F.S., Shankweiler, D.P., Studdert-Kennedy, M. 1967. Perception of the speech code. Psychol Rev 74, 431–461.

Liberman, M.C., Dodds, L.W., Pierce, S. 1990. Afferent and efferent innervation of the cat cochlea: quantitative analysis with light and electron microscopy. J Comp Neurol 301, 443–460.

Liberman, M.C., Puria, S., Guinan, J.J., Jr. 1996. The ipsilaterally evoked olivocochlear reflex causes rapid adaptation of the $2f_1 - f_2$ distortion product otoacoustic emission. J Acoust Soc Am 99, 3572–3584.

Liberman, M.C., Gao, J., He, D.Z., Wu, X., Jia, S., Zuo, J. 2002. Prestin is required for electromotility of the outer hair cell and for the cochlear amplifier. Nature 419, 300–304.

Liebenthal, E., Binder, J.R., Spitzer, S.M., Possing, E.T., Medler, D.A. 2005. Neural substrates of phonemic perception. Cereb Cortex 15, 1621–1631.

Liégeois-Chauvel, C., de Graaf, J.B., Laguitton, V., Chauvel, P. 1999. Specialization of left auditory cortex for speech perception in man depends on temporal coding. Cereb Cortex 9, 484–496.

Lim, D.J. 1986. Effects of noise and ototoxic drugs at the cellular level in the cochlea: a review. Am J Otolaryngol 7, 73–99.

Lim, K.M., Steele, C.R. 2002. A three-dimensional nonlinear active cochlear model analyzed by the WKB-numeric method. Hear Res 170, 190–205.

Limb, C.J. 2006. Structural and functional neural correlates of music perception. Anat Rec A Discov Mol Cell Evol Biol 288, 435–446.

Liu, W., Suga, N. 1997. Binaural and commissural organization of the primary auditory cortex of the mustached bat. J Comp Physiol [A] 181, 599–605.

Loftus, W.C., Sutter, M.L. 2001. Spectrotemporal organization of excitatory and inhibitory receptive fields of cat posterior auditory field neurons. J Neurophysiol 86, 475–491.

Loftus, W.C., Bishop, D.C., Saint Marie, R.L., Oliver, D.L. 2004. Organization of binaural excitatory and inhibitory inputs to the inferior colliculus from the superior olive. J Comp Neurol 472, 330–344.

Lohuis, T.D., Fuzessery, Z.M. 2000. Neuronal sensitivity to interaural time differences in the sound envelope in the auditory cortex of the pallid bat. Hear Res 143, 43–57.

Lomber, S.G., Malhotra, S., Hall, A.J. 2007. Functional specialization in non-primary auditory cortex of the cat: areal and laminar contributions to sound localization. Hear Res 229, 31–45.

Löwenheim, H., Furness, D.N., Kil, J., Zinn, C., Gultig, K., Fero, M.L., Frost, D., Gummer, A.W., Roberts, J.M., Rubel, E.W., Hackney, C.M., Zenner, H.P. 1999. Gene disruption of p27(Kip1) allows cell proliferation in the postnatal and adult organ of Corti. Proc Natl Acad Sci USA 96, 4084–4088.

Löwenstein, O., Wersäll, J. 1959. A functional interpretation of the electron-microscopic structure of sensory hairs in the cristae of the elasmobranch Raja clavata in terms of directional sensitivity. Nature 184, 1807–1808.

Lu, T.K., Zhak, S., Dallos, P., Sarpeshkar, R. 2006. Fast cochlear amplification with slow outer hair cells. Hear Res 214, 45–67.

Lumpkin, E.A., Hudspeth, A.J. 1995. Detection of Ca^{2+} entry through mechanosensitive channels localizes the site of mechanoelectrical transduction in hair cells. Proc Natl Acad Sci USA 92, 10297–301.

Lustig, L.R. 2006. Nicotinic acetylcholine receptor structure and function in the efferent auditory system. Anat Rec A Discov Mol Cell Evol Biol 288, 424–434.

Lynch, E.D., Kil, J. 2005. Compounds for the prevention and treatment of noise-induced hearing loss. Drug Discov Today 10, 1291–1298.

Lynch, T.J., Nedzelnitsky, V., Peake, W.T. 1982. Input impedance of the cochlea in cat. J Acoust Soc Am 72, 108–130.

Ma, X., Suga, N. 2001. Plasticity of bat's central auditory system evoked by focal electric stimulation of auditory and/or somatosensory cortices. J Neurophysiol 85, 1078–1087.

Maiorana, C.R., Staecker, H. 2005. Advances in inner ear gene therapy: exploring cochlear protection and regeneration. Curr Opin Otolaryngol Head Neck Surg 13, 308–312.

Maison, S., Micheyl, C., Collet, L. 2001. Influence of focused auditory attention on cochlear activity in humans. Psychophysiology 38, 35–40.

Maison, S.F., Luebke, A.E., Liberman, M.C., Zuo, J. 2002. Efferent protection from acoustic injury is mediated via alpha9 nicotinic acetylcholine receptors on outer hair cells. J Neurosci 22, 10838–10846.

Maison, S.F., Adams, J.C., Liberman, M.C. 2003a. Olivocochlear innervation in the mouse: immunocytochemical maps, crossed versus uncrossed contributions, and transmitter colocalization. J Comp Neurol 455, 406–416.

Maison, S.F., Emeson, R.B., Adams, J.C., Luebke, A.E., Liberman, M.C. 2003b. Loss of alpha CGRP reduces sound-evoked activity in the cochlear nerve. J Neurophysiol 90, 2941–2949.

Maison, S.F., Rosahl, T.W., Homanics, G.E., Liberman, M.C. 2006. Functional role of GABAergic innervation of the cochlea: phenotypic analysis of mice lacking GABA(A) receptor subunits alpha 1, alpha 2, alpha 5, alpha 6, beta 2, beta 3, or delta. J Neurosci 26, 10315–10326.

Maison, S.F., Parker, L.L., Young, L., Adelman, J.P., Zuo, J., Liberman, M.C. 2007. Overexpression of SK2 channels enhances efferent suppression of cochlear responses without enhancing noise resistance. J Neurophysiol 97, 2930–2936.

Majewska, A.K., Sur, M. 2006. Plasticity and specificity of cortical processing networks. Trends Neurosci 29, 323–329.

Malhotra, S., Lomber, S.G. 2007. Sound localization during homotopic and heterotopic bilateral cooling deactivation of primary and nonprimary auditory cortical areas in the cat. J Neurophysiol 97, 26–43.

Malhotra, S., Hall, A.J., Lomber, S.G. 2004. Cortical control of sound localization in the cat: unilateral cooling deactivation of 19 cerebral areas. J Neurophysiol 92, 1625–1643.

Malmierca, M.S., Leergaard, T.B., Bajo, V.M., Bjaalie, J.G., Merchan, M.A. 1998. Anatomic evidence of a three-dimensional mosaic pattern of tonotopic organization in the ventral complex of the lateral lemniscus in cat. J Neurosci 18, 10603–10618.

Malmierca, M.S., Merchan, M.A., Henkel, C.K., Oliver, D.L. 2002. Direct projections from cochlear nuclear complex to auditory thalamus in the rat. J Neurosci 22, 10891–10897.

Mammano, F., Ashmore, J.F. 1993. Reverse transduction measured in the isolated cochlea by laser Michelson interferometry. Nature 365, 838–841.

Marcus, D.C., Wu, T., Wangemann, P., Kofuji, P. 2002. KCNJ10 (Kir4.1) potassium channel knockout abolishes endocochlear potential. Am J Physiol Cell Physiol 282, C403–C407.

Maren, S., Quirk, G.J. 2004. Neuronal signalling of fear memory. Nat Rev Neurosci 5, 844–52.

Markin, V.S., Hudspeth, A.J. 1995. Gating-spring models of mechanoelectrical transduction by hair cells of the internal ear. Annu Rev Biophys Biomol Struct 24, 59–83.

Martin, R.C. 2003. Language processing: functional organization and neuroanatomical basis. Annu Rev Psychol 54, 55–89.

Martin, P., Bozovic, D., Choe, Y., Hudspeth, A.J. 2003. Spontaneous oscillation by hair bundles of the bullfrog's sacculus. J Neurosci 23, 4533–4548.

Masterton, B., Diamond, I.T. 1967. Medial superior olive and sound localization. Science 155, 1696–1697.

Matsubara, J.A., Phillips, D.P. 1988. Intracortical connections and their physiological correlates in the primary auditory cortex (AI) of the cat. J Comp Neurol 268, 38–48.

Matsui, J.I., Ryals, B.M. 2005. Hair cell regeneration: an exciting phenomenon . . . But will restoring hearing and balance be possible? J Rehabil Res Dev 42, 187–198.

Matsumoto, N., Kalinec, F. 2005. Prestin-dependent and prestin-independent motility of guinea pig outer hair cells. Hear Res 208, 1–13.

May, B.J. 2000. Role of the dorsal cochlear nucleus in the sound localization behavior of cats. Hear Res 148, 74–87.

May, B.J., Prell, G.S., Sachs, M.B. 1998. Vowel representations in the ventral cochlear nucleus of the cat: effects of level, background noise, and behavioral state. J Neurophysiol 79, 1755–1767.

McAlpine, D. 2005. Creating a sense of auditory space. J Physiol 566, 21–28.

McAlpine, D., Palmer, A.R. 2002. Blocking GABAergic inhibition increases sensitivity to sound motion cues in the inferior colliculus. J Neurosci 22, 1443–1453.

McAlpine, D., Jiang, D., Palmer, A.R. 2001. A neural code for low-frequency sound localization in mammals. Nat Neurosci 4, 396–401.

McBride, D.I., Williams, S. 2001. Audiometric notch as a sign of noise induced hearing loss. Occup Environ Med 58, 46–51.

Spoendlin, H. 1978. The afferent innervation of the cochlea. In: Naunton, R.F., Fernandez, C. (Eds), Evoked Electrical Activity in the Auditory Nervous System. Academic Press, London. pp. 21–39.

Sridhar, D., Stakhovskaya, O., Leake, P.A. 2006. A frequency-position function for the human cochlear spiral ganglion. Audiol Neurootol 11 Suppl 1, 16–20.

Srinivasan, G., Friauf, E., Lohrke, S. 2004. Functional glutamatergic and glycinergic inputs to several superior olivary nuclei of the rat revealed by optical imaging. Neuroscience 128, 617–634.

Stecker, G.C., Mickey, B.J., Macpherson, E.A., Middlebrooks, J.C. 2003. Spatial sensitivity in field PAF of cat auditory cortex. J Neurophysiol 89, 2889–2903.

Stecker, G.C., Harrington, I.A., Macpherson, E.A., Middlebrooks, J.C. 2005. Spatial sensitivity in the dorsal zone (area DZ) of cat auditory cortex. J Neurophysiol 94, 1267–1280.

Sterkers, O., Ferrary, E., Amiel, C. 1984. Inter- and intracompartmental osmotic gradients within the rat cochlea. Am J Physiol 247, F602–F606.

Stewart, L., von Kriegstein, K., Warren, J.D., Griffiths, T.D. 2006. Music and the brain: disorders of musical listening. Brain 129, 2533–2553.

Stone, J.S., Cotanche, D.A. 2007. Hair cell regeneration in the avian auditory epithelium. Int J Dev Biol 51, 633–647.

Suga, N., Ma, X. 2003. Multiparametric corticofugal modulation and plasticity in the auditory system. Nat Rev Neurosci 4, 783–794.

Suga, N., Zhang, Y., Yan, J. 1997. Sharpening of frequency tuning by inhibition in the thalamic auditory nucleus of the mustached bat. J Neurophysiol 77, 2098–2114.

Sukharev, S., Corey, D.P. 2004. Mechanosensitive channels: multiplicity of families and gating paradigms. Sci STKE 2004, 219, re4.

Sutherland, D.P., Masterton, R.B., Glendenning, K.K. 1998a. Role of acoustic striae in hearing: reflexive responses to elevated sound-sources. Behav Brain Res 97, 1–12.

Sutherland, D.P., Glendenning, K.K., Masterton, R.B. 1998b. Role of acoustic striae in hearing: discrimination of sound-source elevation. Hear Res 120, 86–108.

Sutter, M.L., Schreiner, C.E. 1991. Physiology and topography of neurons with multipeaked tuning curves in cat primary auditory cortex. J Neurophysiol 65, 1207–1226.

Sutter, M.L., Schreiner, C.E., McLean, M., O'Connor K.N., Loftus, W.C. 1999. Organization of inhibitory frequency receptive fields in cat primary auditory cortex. J Neurophysiol 82, 2358–2371.

Sweet, R.A., Dorph-Petersen, K.A., Lewis, D.A. 2005. Mapping auditory core, lateral belt, and parabelt cortices in the human superior temporal gyrus. J Comp Neurol 491, 270–289.

Talavage, T.M., Sereno, M.I., Melcher, J.R., Ledden, P.J., Rosen, B.R., Dale, A.M. 2004. Tonotopic organization in human auditory cortex revealed by progressions of frequency sensitivity. J Neurophysiol 91, 1282–1296.

Talwar, S.K., Musial, P.G., Gerstein, G.L. 2001. Role of mammalian auditory cortex in the perception of elementary sound properties. J Neurophysiol 85, 2350–2358.

Tan, Q., Carney, L.H. 2006. Predictions of formant-frequency discrimination in noise based on model auditory-nerve responses. J Acoust Soc Am 120, 1435–1445.

Tanaka, M., Yoshida, M., Emoto, H., Ishii, H. 2000. Noradrenaline systems in the hypothalamus, amygdala and locus coeruleus are involved in the provocation of anxiety: basic studies. Eur J Pharmacol 405, 397–406.

Tasaki, I. 1954. Nerve impulses in individual auditory nerve fibers of guinea pig. J Neurophysiol 17, 97–122.

Tasaki, I., Spyropoulos, C.S. 1959. Stria vascularis as source of endocochlear potential. J Neurophysiol 22, 149–155.

Tasaki, I., Davis, H., Legouix, J.P. 1952. The space-time pattern of the cochlear microphonics (guinea pig), as recorded by differential electrodes. J Acoust Soc Am 24, 502–519.

Tasaki, I., Davis, H., Eldredge, D.H. 1954. Exploration of cochlear potentials in guinea pig with a microelectrode. J Acoust Soc Am 26, 765–773.

Tateya, I., Nakagawa, T., Iguchi, F., Kim, T.S., Endo, T., Yamada, S., Kageyama, R., Naito, Y., Ito, J. 2003. Fate of neural stem cells grafted into injured inner ears of mice. Neuroreport 14, 1677–1681.

Temchin, A.N., Rich, N.C., Ruggero, M.A. 1997. Low-frequency suppression of auditory nerve responses to characteristic frequency tones. Hear Res 113, 29–56.

Thierry, G., Giraud, A.L., Price, C. 2003. Hemispheric dissociation in access to the human semantic system. Neuron 38, 499–506.

Thompson, A.M. 2003a. A medullary source of norepinephrine in cat cochlear nuclear complex. Exp Brain Res 153, 486–490.

Thompson, A.M. 2003b. Pontine sources of norepinephrine in the cat cochlear nucleus. J Comp Neurol 457, 374–383.

Thompson, G.C., Masterton, R.B. 1978. Brain stem auditory pathways involved in reflexive head orientation to sound. J Neurophysiol 41, 1183–1202.

Thornton, S.K., Withington, D.J. 1996. The role of the external nucleus of the inferior colliculus in the construction of the superior collicular auditory space map in the guinea-pig. Neurosci Res 25, 239–246.

Tian, B., Rauschecker, J.P. 1994. Processing of frequency-modulated sounds in the cat's anterior auditory field. J Neurophysiol 71, 1959–1975.

Tian, B., Rauschecker, J.P. 1998. Processing of frequency-modulated sounds in the cat's posterior auditory field. J Neurophysiol 79, 2629–2642.

Tian, B., Rauschecker, J.P. 2004. Processing of frequency-modulated sounds in the lateral auditory belt cortex of the rhesus monkey. J Neurophysiol 92, 2993–3013.

Tian, B., Reser, D., Durham, A., Kustov, A., Rauschecker, J.P. 2001. Functional specialization in rhesus monkey auditory cortex. Science 292, 290–293.

Tilney, L.G., Derosier, D.J., Mulroy, M.J. 1980. The organization of actin filaments in the stereocilia of cochlear hair cells. J Cell Biol 86, 244–259.

Tilney, L.G., Saunders, J.C., Egelman, E., DeRosier, D.J. 1982. Changes in the organization of actin filaments in the stereocilia of noise-damaged lizard cochleae. Hear Res 7, 181–197.

Tollin, D.J., Yin, T.C. 2002. The coding of spatial location by single units in the lateral superior olive of the cat. II. The determinants of spatial receptive fields in azimuth. J Neurosci 22, 1468–1479.

Tollin, D.J., Yin, T.C. 2005. Interaural phase and level difference sensitivity in low-frequency neurons in the lateral superior olive. J Neurosci 25, 10648–10657.

Tong, Y.C., Blamey, P.J., Dowell, R.C., Clark, G.M. 1983. Psychophysical studies evaluating the feasibility of a speech processing strategy for a multiple-channel cochlear implant. J Acoust Soc Am 74, 73–80.

Trahiotis, C., Bernstein, L.R., Stern, R.M., Buell, T.N. 2005. Interaural correlation as the basis of a working model of binaural processing: an introduction. In: Popper, A.N., Fay, R.R. (Eds), Sound Source Localization, Springer Handbook of Auditory Research, Vol. 25. Springer, New York. pp. 238–271.

Tramo, M.J., Cariani, P.A., Koh, C.K., Makris, N., Braida, L.D. 2005. Neurophysiology and neuroanatomy of pitch perception: auditory cortex. Ann NY Acad Sci 1060, 148–174.

Tsuchitani, C. 1997. Input from the medial nucleus of trapezoid body to an interaural level detector. Hear Res 105, 211–224.

Tsuchitani, C., Boudreau, J.C. 1966. Single unit analysis of cat superior olive S segment with tonal stimuli. J Neurophysiol 29, 684–697.

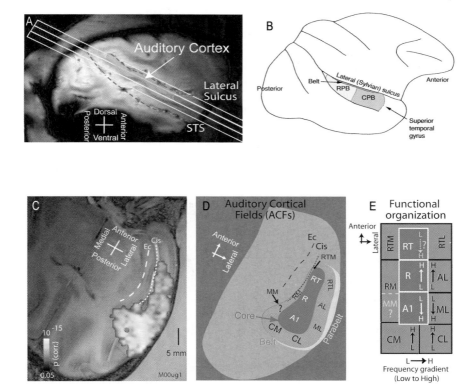

Plate 1 Areas of the monkey (macaque) right auditory cortex as shown by functional magnetic resonance imaging (fMRI). fMRI uses the response to changes in intense magnetic fields to detect activity-related changes in the oxygen depletion of blood. (A) Side view of cortex, showing the planes, through the lower edge of the lateral sulcus, over which images were taken. (B) Diagrammatic representation of the macaque cortex from the same point of view as in part A. The rostral and caudal parabelt areas (RPB, CPB) are shown on the surface of the superior temporal gyrus. (C) Response to broadband noise in one animal. (D) The three core auditory areas (blue) are surrounded by eight belt areas. (E) Tonotopicity of the three core areas and four of the belt areas, shown by representation of high (H) and low (L) frequencies. A1, primary auditory area; AL, anterolateral area; Cis, circular sulcus; CL, caudolateral area; CM, caudomedian area; CPB, caudal parabelt; Ec, external capsule; ML, middle lateral area; MM, middle medial area; R, rostral area; RM, rostromedial area; RPB, rostral parabelt; RT, rostrotemporal area; RTL, lateral rostrotemporal area; RTM, medial rostrotemporal area; STS, superior temporal sulcus. Figure 7.2A, C–E from Petkov *et al.* (2006), Fig. 2. (See Fig. 7.2, p. 211).

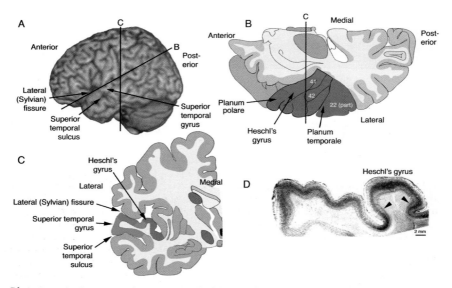

Plate 2 The human auditory cortex (left hemisphere). (A) Lateral view of left cerebral hemisphere, showing planes of section in parts B and C. (B) Sloping section in the plane shown in part A. Top view of upper surface of temporal lobe (red) with area of koniocortex within Heschl's gyrus marked (darker red). The division of the surface anterior to Heschl's gyrus is known as the planum polare, and the large division posterior to Heschl's gyrus is known as the planum temporale. Numbers show areas according to Brodmann (1909). In some individuals, Heschl's gyrus divides into two. (C) Transverse section of left cerebral hemisphere in the vertical plane shown in part A, showing Heschl's gyrus (darker red) and further auditory cortex of the superior temporal plane (lighter red, lighter and darker blue). Exactly how the latter areas are distributed over the superior temporal gyrus and sulcus varies between individuals. (D) Transverse histological section as in part C, showing Heschl's gyrus and laterally adjacent parts of the superior temporal plane. Arrowheads: borders of AI. Nissl stain.

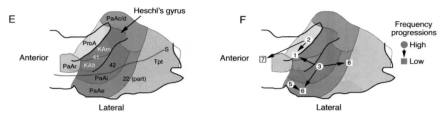

Plate 2 (Continued) (E) Cytoarchitectonic areas of the human auditory cortex according to Galaburda and Sanides (1980). The dotted line (S) shows the position of the Sylvian sulcus: the cortical surface lateral to this line curves down over the external surface of the temporal lobe, over the superior temporal gyrus. The area corresponds to coloured area in part B and extending slightly more anteriorly and further laterally over the superior temporal gyrus. Numbers show areas according to Brodmann (1909). (F) Tonotopic frequency progressions in the cortex, according to Talavage *et al.* (2004), superimposed on the cytoarchitectonic areas of Galaburda and Sanides. The arrows mark the direction of the progressions from high frequency to low. KAlt, lateral koniocortex; KAm, medial koniocortex, PaAc/d: caudo-dorsal parakoniocortex; PaAe, external parakoniocortex; PaAi, internal parakoniocortex; PaAr, rostral parakoniocortex; ProA, prokoniocortex; S, Sylvian (lateral) sulcus or fissure; Tpt, temporoparietal area. Figure 7.4B and C reprinted from Harasty *et al.* (2003), Figure 1, with permission of Taylor and Francis Ltd (http://www.informaworld.com); Figure 7.4D from Wallace *et al.* (2002), Fig. 1A, with kind permission from Springer Science and Business Media; Figure 7.4E and F used with permission from Talavage *et al.* (2004), Fig. 7. (See Fig. 7.4, p. 213, 214).